D0265836

Client Profiles in Nursing

Adult and
the Elderly 2

WITHDRAWN

LANCHESTER LIBRARY, Coventry University
Gosford Street, Coventry CVI 5DD Telephone 024 7688 7555

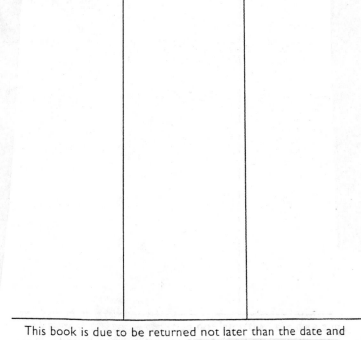

This book is due to be returned not later than the date and
time stamped above. Fines are charged on overdue books

Client Profiles in Nursing

Adult and the Elderly 2

Edited by

S Parboteeah PhD MSc SRN Dip N RCNT Cert Ed

Senior Lecturer
School of Nursing and Midwifery
De Montfort University
Leicester

P Tremayne MSc PGDE BSc (Hons) Dip N RGN

Senior Lecturer
School of Nursing and Midwifery
De Montfort University
Leicester

Lanchester Library

WITHDRAWN

www.greenwich-medical.co.uk

© 2003
Greenwich Medical Media Limited
137 Euston Road
London
NW1 2AA

870 Market Street, Ste 720
San Francisco
CA 94102

ISBN 1 84110 150 8

First published 2003

While the advice and information in this book is believed to be true and accurate, neither the authors nor the publisher can accept any legal responsibility or liability for any loss or damage arising from actions or decisions based in this book. The ultimate responsibility for the treatment of patients and the interpretation lies with the medical practitioner. The opinions expressed are those of the authors and the inclusion in this book of information relating to a particular product, method or technique does not amount to an endorsement of its value or quality, or of the claims made by its manufacturer. Every effort has been made to check drug dosages; however, it is still possible that errors have occurred. Furthermore, dosage schedules are constantly being revised and new side-effects recognised. For these reasons, the medical practitioner is strongly urged to consult the drug companies' printed instructions before administering any of the drugs mentioned in this book.

Apart from any fair dealing for the purposes of research or private study, or criticism or review, as permitted under the UK Copyright Designs and Patents Act 1988, this publication may not be reproduced, stored, or transmitted, in any form or by any means, without the prior permission in writing of the publishers, or in the case of reprographic reproduction only in accordance with the terms of the licences issued by the appropriate Reproduction Rights Organisations outside the UK. Enquiries concerning reproduction outside the terms stated here should be sent to the publishers at the London address printed above.

The rights of Sam Parboteeah and Penny Tremayne to be identified as editors of this work has been asserted by them in accordance with the Copyright Designs and Patents Act 1988.

The publisher makes no representation, express or implied, with regard to the accuracy of the information contained in this book and cannot accept any legal responsibility or liability for any errors or omissions that may be made.

A catalogue record for this book is available from the British Library.

Distributed by Plymbridge Distributors, UK and in the USA by Jamco Distribution

Typeset by Mizpah Publishing Services, Chennai, India
Printed in the UK by the Alden Group, Oxford

Coventry University

Contents

This volume has been designed to be utilised as a study guide for students undertaking health related courses and as a teaching aid for lecturers using a problem based approach to developing professional knowledge and competence. It has a number of classic client profiles that practitioners frequently encounter within the adult and elderly practice setting.

Each profile has been written by a subject specialist and this approach has enabled each case to be embedded in the reality of clinical practice, reflecting an evidence based methodology to managing care. The originality of the cases should stimulate discussion in relation to contemporary practice. Although, some of the cases may appear complex, students and professionals alike can readily identify and recognise their own practice within it.

Each case brings together into a coherent framework the relationship between theory and practice. It is envisaged that the student will gain knowledge and understanding of the issues that most commonly present in relation to the client profile, for example, pathophysiology, medical and nursing interventions and psychosocial issues. However, the format for case 37 differs; the author describes an experience and the reader is asked to reflect on their own practice.

The diversity of the client profiles is indicative of the range and background of the contributing authors. This volume focuses on the nursing of adults and the elderly and there has been a deliberate attempt to present a range of ethnic backgrounds, gender, social status, as well as acute and chronic conditions reflecting nursing in a multicultural society.

Each profile takes the familiar format of a scenario, posing of questions, answers and a reference list including relevant web sites and addresses. It is intended that this volume is used in a dynamic way and can facilitate the following:

- Independent study
- A problem solving approach to care
- Act as a revision aid
- Link theory to practice
- An additional resource for lecturers and practitioners

We hope the reader finds these client profiles relevant and useful in their practice.

Sam Parboteeah
Penny Tremayne
April 2003

Ricky Autar, PhD, MSc, BA (Hons) RGN, RMN, Dip N, Cert Ed.
Principal Lecturer
School of Nursing and Midwifery
De Montfort University
Leicester

Julia Ball, SRN
Ward Sister Gastro-Intestinal Surgery
Leicester General Hospital
Leicester

Chris Buswell
Freelance Nurse Writer
Aberdeenshire

Maggie Chappell, RGN
Public Health Nurse Tuberculosis
Northampton NHS Primary Care Trust
Northampton

Penny Harrison, MA, BSc (Hons), RGN, Cert Ed.
Senior Lecturer
School of Nursing and Midwifery
De Montfort University
Leicester

Kim Leong, MA, RGN, RCNT, Cert Ed.
Senior Lecturer
St Martin's College
Lancaster

Abigail Moriarty, MEd, PGDE, BSc
Senior Lecturer
School of Nursing and Midwifery
De Montfort University
Leicester

Sam Parboteeah, PhD, MSc, SRN, Dip N, RCNT, Cert Ed.
Senior Lecturer
School of Nursing and Midwifery
De Montfort University
Leicester

Danny Pertab, MSc, BSc (Hons), PGCEA, RGN
Senior Lecturer
School of Nursing and Midwifery
De Montfort University
Leicester

Lynn Randall, BSc (Hons), Dip Health Studies, RGN, Cert Ed. Cert HSM
Practice Development Educator
Cardiac Intensive Care Unit
Glenfield Hospital
Leicester

Carolyn Reid, BSc (Hons), RGN
Transplant Coordinator and Practice Educator
Intensive Therapy Unit
Aberdeen Royal Infirmary
Aberdeen

Liz Shears, MA, BA (Hons), RGN, RCNT, Dip N
Senior Lecturer
School of Nursing and Midwifery
De Montfort University
Leicester

Penny Tremayne, MSc, PGDE, BSc (Hons), Dip N, RGN
Senior Lecturer
School of Nursing and Midwifery
De Montfort University
Leicester

Acknowledgement

We are grateful to all the authors for their contributions and the Series Editor for guidance.

Unstable angina

Penny Tremayne

> Geoffrey Ellis is a 50-year-old financial advisor for a bank who lives with his wife, Jenny in a semi-detached house. They have two sons, Lawrence a 19-year-old first year university student and 15-year-old Neil who is preparing to sit end of year examinations.
>
> Currently Jenny who normally works part-time in a hairdressing salon is recuperating after undergoing abdominal surgery.
>
> Over recent months Geoffrey has worked long hours, commuting lengthy distances by car to keep appointments with other branch offices. Often his day involves leaving home by 7.00 a.m. and returning between 7.00 and 9.00 p.m. In his spare time Geoffrey enjoys walking the family dog and is a referee for a local junior school football league.
>
> Geoffrey successfully gave up smoking five years ago having started in his early teens. He enjoys wine and beer and drinks 35 units a week (usual limit is 28 units a week). Due to his busy schedule, the timing of his meals has become irregular and Geoffrey has been opting to eat more convenience fast foods.
>
> Geoffrey has noticed that he is becoming increasingly short of breath on exertion and has experienced occasional chest pain. This has usually been relieved by rest. However, whilst mowing the lawn, Geoffrey experiences a severe tightness in the chest and shortness of breath. Neither rest nor commonly used pain killers are effective and therefore Neil phones for the ambulance.
>
> Geoffrey is admitted to the local hospital where the medical team make a provisional diagnosis of unstable angina pectoris. On admission to hospital his pulse, respiratory rate and blood pressure (BP) are above normal limits and oxygen saturation is 91%.

Question one: What is angina pectoris? Explain the difference between stable and unstable angina.

10 minutes

Question two: Explain the immediate nursing and medical interventions that Geoffrey will require on admission to hospital.

25 minutes

Question three: Discuss the advice that Geoffrey will require on discharge.

15 minutes

Time allowance: **50 minutes**

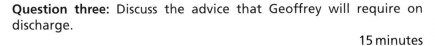

Answer to question one:
What is angina pectoris? Explain the difference between stable and unstable angina.

Angina pectoris is a medical condition that presents itself because of a reduction in the arterial blood supply to the myocardial heart muscle. This can be attributed to:

- Atheromatous plaques causing gradual, progressive narrowing of the coronary arteries
- Partial thrombus formation causing a more sudden, rapid narrowing of the coronary arteries.

Department of Health (2000)

Stable angina can be described as symptoms that remain unchanged or progress slowly. Pain brought on by physical exertion is either relieved by medication or rest.

Unstable angina can be described as severe, prolonged symptoms (lasting more than 15–20 minutes) that occur at night or at rest. These symptoms can advance rapidly and could progress to early death, myocardial infarction or refractory angina (Department of Health, 2000).

Answer to question two:
Explain the immediate nursing and medical interventions that Geoffrey will require on admission to hospital.

General measures of nursing care will include initial bed rest (Department of Health, 2000; Docherty, 2001) and being nursed in an area in which he will be easily observed. Resuscitation equipment should be close to hand. Geoffrey's heart rate should be observed continuously by placing chest leads and attaching to a cardiac monitor. To improve myocardial oxygen supply, 28% oxygen may be prescribed and administered.

The extent of Geoffrey's chest pain should be identified by using an assessment tool (Standing, 1997) and by actively listening to what the patient is saying (Albarran, 2002). Initially, pain relief may be achieved by nitrate therapy (either intravenously if the pain is recurring or sublingually for short, episodic pain).

Geoffrey should be informed that he may experience a headache or some flushing after taking a sublingual nitrate. In the event of the pain being very severe, then diamorphine intravenously 2.5–5 mg may be prescribed and repeated until pain is relieved alongside an appropriate anti-emetic. An electrocardiogram (ECG) should be recorded, and if symptoms continue or if he complains of further chest pain, then subsequent ECGs should be recorded to monitor for possible ischaemic changes (ST segment depression, T wave inversion or flattened T wave).

Monitoring will include: temperature, pulse, respiratory rate, oxygen saturation, blood pressure. The following blood tests will be performed: electrolyte levels, fasting total serum cholesterol (will be measured at some 12–24 hours post admission), a serum troponin-T level (will be taken to identify if there is any myocardial damage).

Geoffrey will receive anti-thrombolytic therapy. This can include aspirin 300 mg (Department of Health, 2000) and either intravenous heparin or more usually a low molecular subcutaneous heparin which is given for up to 2–5 days, until pain free. A daily maintenance dose of 75–150 mg aspirin is usually prescribed.

Anti-ischaemic drugs such as beta-blockers have long been the first choice to lower the resting heart rate and BP to less than 140/85 mmHg (Department of Health, 2000). Examples of beta-blockers such as atenolol and metoprolol have side effects which include: tiredness, cold extremities, insomnia, and bronchospasm. Mead (1998) and MacDermott (2001) caution that such agents should be used with caution in patients who have heart failure, peripheral vascular disease and diabetes and is contraindicated in those with asthma. Long-acting nitrates are often used in combination with beta-blockers. Examples include isosorbide dinitrate and isosorbide mononitrate. Side effects include headache and flushing and tolerance becomes less effective after prolonged use (Mead, 1998).

Reserved for second or third line therapy or when beta-blockers are contraindicated, calcium antagonists like verapamil or diltiazem may be used. Side effects include headache, flushing and ankle swelling (Mead, 1998). Geoffrey may also be a candidate for future revascularisation (angioplasty, coronary artery bypass graft); this can reduce the risk of death or future cardiac events (Department of Health, 2000).

Depending on the result of the fasting total serum cholesterol and aiming to reduce the serum cholesterol concentration to less than 5 mmol or a reduction of 30% whichever is the greater (Department of Health, 2000; MacDermott, 2001), Geoffrey may also be commenced on a lipid lowering statin therapy.

It is important that whilst all these acute interventions are occurring that the nurse has an ongoing dialogue with Geoffrey and his family, informing him/them about what is happening and why. Albarran (2002) highlights that it is important that nurses actively listen as this not only gives the patient the opportunity to interpret their experience but it can also convey empathy. This will hopefully contribute to a reduction in the anxiety that Geoffrey will be experiencing.

Answer to question three:
Discuss the advice that Geoffrey will require on discharge.

Now the angina is stable, and before discharge from hospital, Geoffrey will be referred for the first phase of cardiac rehabilitation (Department of Health, 2000). This phase comprises of:

- Assessment of physical needs, namely desirable lifestyle (increased physical activity, smoking cessation, diet, alcohol consumption, medication and further clinical management), educational (provide information about what to do should similar or more severe symptoms reoccur), psychological and social, cultural, vocational, family needs
- Formation of a negotiated plan to include an individualised exercise regimen, counselling, education, stress reduction
- Initial advice on lifestyle: physical activity (including sexual activity), diet, alcohol consumption and employment
- Prescription of effective medication and education about its use, storage, benefits and side effects
- Advice on how to deal with future similar episodes
- Involvement of family members as necessary and as able
- Provision of information about cardiac support groups
- Provision of relevant information leaflets.

References

Albarran, J. (2002) The language of chest pain. Nursing Times 98(4): 38–40.
Department of Health (2000) National Service Framework for Coronary Heart Disease: Modern standards and service models. London: The Stationery Office.
Docherty, B. (2001) Chest pain management. Professional Nurse 16(9): 1334–1335.
MacDermott, A. (2001) Approaches to improving outcome in stable angina. Professional Nurse 16(8): 1302–1305.
Mead, M. (1998) Drugs for angina. Practice Nurse 15(4): 220–221.
Standing, J. (1997) Chest pain assessment tools. Journal of Clinical Nursing 6(2): 85–92.

Suggested reading

Landowski, R., Sulman, R., Davies, R. (2002) Drugs Used in Heart Disease: 1. Pharmacology. Nursing Times 98(18): 43–46.
Sulman, R., Davies, R., Landowski, R. (2002) Drugs Used in Heart Disease: 2. Pharmacology. Nursing Times 98(18): 41–44.

Useful addresses

British Association for Cardiac Rehabilitation
9 Fitzroy Square,
London
W1T 5HW
Tel: 020 73833887
Website: www.bcs.com/bacr

British Heart Foundation,
14 Fitzhardinge Street,
London
W1H 6DH
Tel: 020 79350185
Website: www.bhf.org.uk

Crohn's disease

Penny Harrison

Sue Stanley a 38-year-old primary school teacher, is single, but sees her boyfriend at weekends, as he lives in the neighbouring city and works away during the week. Sue has her own room in a terraced house which she shares with a work colleague and a friend. There is one small bathroom with a shower, but not a bath. Sue and her two house mates share the living accommodation downstairs.

When Sue is in good health, she maintains a full and busy social life, often going out with friends to the cinema during the week in the evenings. She smokes 10 cigarettes a day. She does not drink during the week, but admits to drinking 20 units of alcohol when out with her boyfriend most Saturday nights, especially when they enjoy a meal out. Her family live close by and Sue baby sits for her sister's children each Wednesday, collecting the four children en route home from work, preparing their supper and putting them to bed.

Sue has been diagnosed with Crohn's disease since she was 22. She is usually in reasonable health, with a medication regimen of Pentasa 500 mg three times daily. However, during the last 2 years, Sue has had increasing exacerbations of her Crohn's disease, usually a 2–3 week episode every 3 months. Sue is then off sick from work whilst hospitalised and for up to 2 weeks post discharge as she convalesces. The symptoms of her exacerbations are abdominal pain, frequent episodes of diarrhoea, passing soft watery stools that contain mucous, hyper pyrexia, nausea and sometimes episodes of vomiting. During these periods of ill health, Sue can lose between 8 and 12 kg in weight (Sue's usual weight is 50 kg). On two previous occasions, Sue has been hospitalised, requiring intravenous fluids and steroids to stabilise her condition. Sue is becoming low in mood and frustrated with her deteriorating health, often reflected in angry outbursts about her treatment to staff on the ward as well as to her family and friends. Sue is finding it increasingly difficult to cope with the demands of her job and states she feels 'guilty' about the amounts of time she is away from work.

Question one: What is Crohn's disease and what factors might contribute to Sue's exacerbations of the disease?

20 minutes

Question two: What treatment is available for Sue during an exacerbation?

20 minutes

Question three: What support can the multi disciplinary team offer Sue to assist with management of her condition?

20 minutes

Time allowance: **60 minutes**

Answer to question one:
What is Crohn's disease and what factors might contribute to Sue's exacerbations of the disease?

Crohn's disease is a disease of the gastrointestinal tract and may affect the tract anywhere from the mouth to the anus. The cause of Crohn's is not known and thus patients require support and management of their symptoms, rather than a cure being available (Metcalf, 2002). It typically affects younger patients from developed countries, with an incidence of 30 to 500 per 100,000 population (Hudson & Goldthorpe, 1997). It is a disease of acute exacerbations or 'flare ups' and remission. The most common site for Crohn's is the terminal ileum (British Society of Gastroenterology, 1996). The entire structure of the lumen of the bowel may be involved, with inflammation spreading to surrounding structures. The symptoms of Crohn's disease are:

- Pain – due to passing of stools via inflamed bowel
- Diarrhoea – rapid transit of blood and or mucous stained stools
- Abnormal blood results – changes to a wide range of immunological blood values
- Anaemia – due to potential deficiencies with iron, vitamin B12 and folate
- Weight loss – due to reduced dietary intake associated with acute exacerbations, and absorption difficulties due to the inflammatory process
- Other inflammatory disorders – such as arthritis and iritis.

There are a range of criteria that are thought to contribute to Crohn's disease. From the profile, an assessment of Sue and her lifestyle might assist the multi disciplinary team to review whether factors were contributing to episodes of acute exacerbation or assisting with remission. Sue could be asked to keep a diary to log life events, dietary intake and record symptoms to assist with this process. Factors that affect Crohn's disease are:

- Diet – Metcalf (2002) suggests that the role of diet in Crohn's disease is complex. For some individuals regulating intake of fibre, sugar and dairy products improves symptoms. Anecdotally, patients are often able to identify food types and products that assist with management of symptoms. What type of foods is Sue likely to eat? At work? Whilst babysitting? When out with her boyfriend?
- Smoking – Kamm (1996) suggests that Crohn's is 2–4 times more common in smokers. Sue smokes 20 cigarettes per day. What factors could the nurse use to inform and advise Sue about the risks of smoking and assist to promote her health?
- Stress – the role of stress in Crohn's is controversial. Metcalf (2002) highlights some studies that have made the link between increased risk of symptom exacerbation and major life stresses such as divorce. What might be Sue's causes of stress? What factors could the nurse employ to assist Sue to manage stress?

Client profiles in nursing: adult & the elderly 2

Answer to question two:
What treatment is available for Sue during an exacerbation?

Treatment for Crohn's disease can be placed into a variety of categories. The nurse has an important role to play in preparing Sue for a variety of tests and investigations. This is to ensure that Sue receives the necessary pre-, during and post-procedure care as well as agreeing and co-operating with the:

Investigations

- Monitoring stool – the nurse maintains a stool chart for recording the date, time, amount, colour, consistency, the presence of blood and mucous.
- Blood tests – the nurse assists the team with the management of symptoms and information gained from blood tests.
- Colonoscopy – the colon is visualised endoscopically, allowing the team to assess the extent and nature of the Crohn's disease affecting the colon. The findings can be used in formulating a plan of treatment.
- Radiological tests – barium studies will assist the team to view Sue's small bowel radiologically. This will allow assessment of the extent and nature of the Crohn's disease that Sue has as well as assisting in the planning of care and treatment.

Treatment for Crohn's disease is two-fold: medical and surgical:

Medical treatment

- Pharmacology – Crohn's disease may be managed by pharmacological treatment. The type and severity of symptoms dictates the range of drugs to be used. Sue is already prescribed an aminosalicylate to manage her disease. The nurse has a key role to play in ensuring that Sue understands the nature of her medications and their role in managing her disease.
- Steroids – may be used to suppress the inflammatory action of the disease process.
- Aminosalicylates – may be used to reduce the inflammation of the bowel locally.
- Antibiotics – antibiotics such as metronidazole may be used as alternatives to aminosalicylates or if there is evidence of infective diarrhoea from stool samples.
- Immunosuppressive therapy – may be used to suppress the inflammatory action of the disease process.
- Anti-diarrhoeal agents – may be used for the relief of symptoms, but have to be used with caution during exacerbation of Crohn's due to the risk of complications.

Medical treatment could also include managing possible anaemia, fluid and electrolyte imbalance, and in severe cases hypovolaemic shock. Transfusion of blood for anaemia (see Case 20 for the responsibilities of the nurse in blood transfusion) or administration of intravenous fluids for correction of dehydration and altered blood chemistry.

Surgical treatment

- Crohn's disease is incurable. Therefore surgical treatment for Crohn's is only indicated for management of complications such as obstruction. This is because diseased bowel may be removed, but other areas of healthy bowel may be affected by the inflammatory process later.

Nutrition

- Nutritional assessment – Sue has a history of weight loss associated with acute exacerbations of her Crohn's disease. The nurse should use a nutritional assessment tool to identify for actual and potential malnutrition. A referral to the dietician may be made for advice if Sue is unable to maintain adequate nutrition.

Answer to question three:
What support can the multi disciplinary team offer Sue to assist with management of her condition?

The nurse is a key individual within the multi disciplinary team to assess, plan and evaluate as well as co-ordinate care. In addition to the nursing and medical staff involved in Sue's care, the team may have a number of other members who offer support and advice. In order to assist Sue to manage her disease, recognition of the role of chronic disease in an individual should not be underestimated. There are a range of issues that patients have to cope with when they have an inflammatory bowel disease such as Crohn's. These are:

- Fatigue – Sue may experience fatigue during an exacerbation of her disease. The nurse can promote a balance of rest and activity, as well as acknowledging that this is not the norm for the individual, but supporting the patient whilst unwell during exacerbation of a chronic disorder.
- Hygiene – When hospitalised Sue should be nursed in a side room with an adjoining toilet. Sue may have to share toilet facilities at work and shares a bathroom at home. The stigma of using the toilet frequently, sometimes urgently whilst making loud noises associated with explosive diarrhoea causes embarrassment and feelings of social stigma and isolation. These symptoms may also limit social activities when Sue is experiencing an acute exacerbation of her disease. The nurse can assist Sue by referring her to a local support group. Sufferers of Crohn's disease may have many practical tips and assistance to be shared in helping Sue to cope with her disease both at work as well as in social situations.
- Body image – Sue may have to undergo a range of intimate investigations such as colonoscopy to monitor her condition. The impact of changes in physical appearance such those caused by exacerbation of the disease (pallor, weight loss) and side effects of drugs such as steroids (facial hair growth) may have an important impact on body image. Sue may view her disease negatively and as having a major affect on her life, as well as influencing relationships with her family, friends or boyfriend.
- Employment – Sue may be concerned about the periods of time she has to take off work when her Crohn's disease is active. The nurse may be able to assist Sue by referring her to the social worker for specialist advice about benefits or payments Sue is entitled to when she is absent from work. A psychologist or counsellor may also be able to provide input with regard to Sue's ability to recognise and manage stress as well.
- Fertility – As Sue is of child bearing age she should seek specialist advice about family planning.

References

British Society of Gastroenterology (1996) Inflammatory Bowel Disease. London: BSG.
Hudson, J., Goldthorpe S. (1997) Chapter 3 'Inflammatory bowel disease' in Bruce, L., Finlay, T.M.D. Nursing in Gastroenterology. New York: Churchill Livingstone.
Kamm, M. (1996) Inflammatory Bowel Disease. London: Martin Dunitz.
Metcalf, C. (2002) Crohn's disease: an overview. Nursing Standard 16(31): 45–52.

Further reading

Bruce, L., Finlay, T. (1997) (Eds) Nursing in Gastroenterology. Edinburgh: Churchill Livingstoné.

Cotton, P., Williams, C. (1996) Practical Gastrointestinal Endoscopy. (4th ed.). Oxford: Blackwell Scientific.

Doughty, D. (1993) Gastroenterology Disorders. St Louis: Mosby.

Hypovolaemic shock

Sam Parboteeah

> Following a road traffic accident (RTA) Eddie O'Connell, a 24-year-old man has been admitted to the Accident and Emergency (A&E) department of the hospital. On arrival, Eddie is able to converse although not orientated to date, time, place or person.
>
> On initial assessment, he appears anxious and his baseline observations are as follows: blood pressure – 80/60 mmHg, a thready pulse – 120 beats per minute, a respiratory rate of 24 breaths per minute, the capillary refill test is slow (>2 s). His extremities are cold and pale.
>
> The paramedic report indicated that Eddie was involved in a collision and that he was trapped in his car. He complained of pain in his left hip and leg area but there are no visible injuries. However, clinical and radiological investigations confirm that Eddie has a fractured left femur (compound fracture).

Question one: Define shock.

5 minutes

Question two: List the signs and symptoms of hypovolaemic shock and discuss how these should be used to assess volume loss in Eddie.

20 minutes

Question three: Discuss the compensatory and haemodynamic changes which occur in response to blood loss.

15 minutes

Question four: Discuss fluid resuscitation and the role of the nurse in monitoring treatment.

20 minutes

Time allowance: **60 minutes**

Answer to question one:
Define shock.

The term shock is used to describe an acute clinical syndrome initiated by hypoperfusion and severe dysfunction of organs. It is a progressive condition of circulatory failure resulting in decreased cardiac output and inadequate delivery of oxygen and nutrients to meet the demands of the body. Because shock involves multiple organs, it can be considered as a systemic disorder and the clinical picture therefore reflects the sum of the effects of each system.

Answer to question two:
List the signs and symptoms of hypovolaemic shock and discuss how these should be used to assess volume loss in Eddie.

Hypovolaemic shock is the commonest type of shock following trauma and the following signs and symptoms are indicative of hypovolaemic shock.

- Hypotension
- Tachycardia
- Reduced pulse pressure
- Skin – pale and cool
- Tachypnoea
- Cyanosis
- Capillary refill test (>2 s) – this involves pressing the nail bed until it becomes blanched, the pressure is then released and the time taken for re-perfusion is less than 2 seconds
- Anxious, aggressive, confused, drowsy, unconscious.

As haemorrhage continues clinical signs and symptoms develop which may be helpful in assessing the volume of blood loss. Baskett (1993) classifies the degree of haemorrhage into four classes:

Class I – There is less than 15% blood loss (750 ml) and this volume of blood loss does not produce any clinical signs (listed above) except for a slight tachycardia. Compensatory mechanism is sufficient to restore blood volume if there is no further blood loss.

Class II – Between 15–30% of blood may be lost (800–1500 ml). There is a rise in diastolic pressure with the systolic pressure remaining normal. The capillary refill test is prolonged (>2 s) and the patient may become anxious or aggressive. The extremities may be cold and pale and the urine volume may be decreased (20–30 ml/h). Fluid replacement is required.

Class III – There is 30–40% blood loss (1500–2000 ml). At this stage compensatory mechanisms fail to restore blood volume. There is hypotension, tachycardia, tachypnoea, pale extremities and complexion. The capillary refill test will be prolonged (>2 s) and the rate of urine flow will be decreased (10–20 ml/h). The patient may be anxious, aggressive or drowsy. This degree of blood volume requires immediate intravenous fluid replacement and blood transfusion in trauma cases. In relation to Eddie's injuries and signs and symptoms this may be the volume of blood that is lost.

Class IV – The volume of blood loss is over 40% (>2000 ml) and can be life threatening. There is a marked degree of hypotension, weak and thready pulse, marked tachycardia, tachypnoea (>20/min). The extremities are cold and pale, and the patient may be confused and drowsy. The capillary refill test becomes undetectable and urine flow is decreased (0–10 ml/h). Management of these patients requires rapid intravenous volume replacement.

Baskett (1993) suggests that the above signs and symptoms are only a guide to volume loss and fluid resuscitation requirements. Thus, fluid replacement must be determined by haemodynamic and other responses rather than being a predetermined estimate of loss. An adequate replacement is indicated by a urine flow of greater than 30 ml/h and a central venous pressure (CVP) which increases 2–3 cmH$_2$O or more in response to a fluid challenge of 250–500 ml.

Answer to question three:
Discuss the compensatory and haemodynamic changes which occur in response to blood loss.

The decrease in blood volume caused by blood loss produces hypotension which results in reduced blood flow to the brain and cardiac muscle. As a result, haemodynamic changes as shown in Figure 3.1 occur, in an attempt to restore an adequate blood circulation.

A second important compensatory mechanism involving capillary fluid exchange results from both the decrease in blood pressure and the increase in arteriolar constrictions both of which decrease capillary hydrostatic pressure thereby favouring absorption of interstitial fluid (Fig. 3.2). Thus, a decrease in blood volume is compensated by the movement of interstitial fluid into the cardiovascular system.

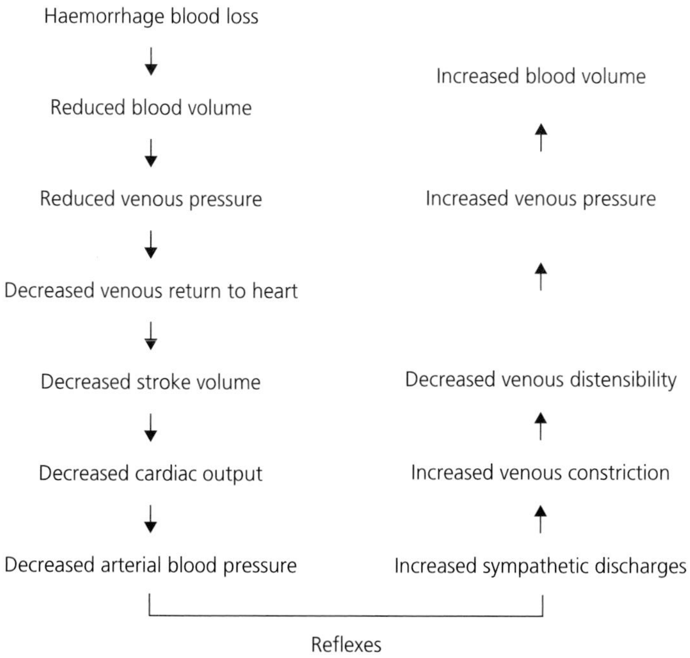

Haemorrhage blood loss
↓
Reduced blood volume
↓
Reduced venous pressure
↓
Decreased venous return to heart
↓
Decreased stroke volume
↓
Decreased cardiac output
↓
Decreased arterial blood pressure

Increased blood volume
↑
Increased venous pressure
↑
Decreased venous distensibility
↑
Increased venous constriction
↑
Increased sympathetic discharges

Reflexes

Figure 3.1: Haemodynamic changes which occur in response to blood loss.

Client profiles in nursing: adult & the elderly 2

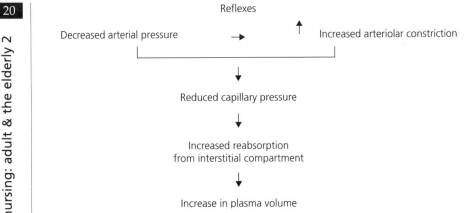

Reflexes

Decreased arterial pressure → ↑ Increased arteriolar constriction

↓

Reduced capillary pressure

↓

Increased reabsorption
from interstitial compartment

↓

Increase in plasma volume

Figure 3.2: Compensatory mechanism involving capillary fluid exchange.

Answer to question four:
Discuss fluid resuscitation and the role of the nurse in monitoring treatment.

Fluid resuscitation for hypovolaemic shock has been the mainstay of medical management of trauma patients. Colloids have been widely used as recommended in a number of resuscitation guidelines and intensive care manuals as plasma substitutes for short term replacement of fluid volume while the problem is being addressed. However, there is continuing uncertainty about the most appropriate fluid. Alderson et al (2002) in their systematic review found no benefit from using colloids over crystalloids.

Whilst the merits of colloids and crystalloids are debated and systematically reviewed as the best blood substitute in hypovolaemic shock, Baskett (1993) suggests that a mixture of colloids and crystalloids provide optimal treatment. He recommends that in severe blood loss (>30% of blood volume) fluid resuscitation should start with colloid (1–1.5l) followed by a litre of crystalloid. Subsequently, equal amount of colloid and crystalloid should be administered until blood is available.

The role of the nurse is two-fold: firstly to administer prescribed fluid regimen and secondly to monitor the effectiveness of fluid resuscitation.

• Administration of fluids and blood products

Even though this is an emergency situation, as a nurse you must always ensure that local policy/protocol is applied.

• Monitoring role

Recording and reporting observation of pulse, blood pressure, skin perfusion, mental state, capillary refill test, respiratory rate, urine flow, CVP (if present) will provide a valuable guide to the status of Eddie's fluid resuscitation.

References

Alderson, P., Schierhout, G., Roberts, I., Bunn, F. (2002) Colloids versus crystalloids for fluid resuscitation in critically ill patients (Cochrane Review). In: The Cochrane Library, issue 1. Oxford: Update Software.
Baskett, P.J.F. (1993) Resuscitation Handbook. London: Wolfe.

Further reading

Bunn, F., Alderson, P., Hawkins, V. (2002) Colloid solutions for fluid resuscitation (Cochrane Review). In: The Cochrane Library, issue 1. Oxford: Update Software.

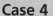

Acute renal failure

Kim Leong

Mrs Rosie Fairhead, aged 69 years old, has recently been widowed. She has three sons living locally. Mrs Fairhead is currently an in-patient in an oncology ward receiving a blood transfusion as her haemoglobin (Hb) level is below normal limits.

Within 20 minutes of starting a second unit of blood Mrs Fairhead complains of pain at the cannula site, abdominal pain, facial flushing. She becomes increasingly more agitated, and reports that she feels unwell. The blood transfusion is stopped immediately and the medical staff informed (for management of transfusion reaction see Case 20).

Whilst monitoring Mrs Fairhead's observations it was noted that she had not passed urine for at least 8 hours which was unusual as she had received diuretics prior to the second unit of blood.

In view of the possible transfusion reaction, it was decided to insert a urethral catheter to ascertain renal function. Later, the doctor informed Mrs Fairhead that she was suffering from acute renal failure.

Question one: Define the term acute renal failure.

5 minutes

Question two: What are the possible causes of acute renal failure?

10 minutes

Question three: What are the pathophysiological manifestations of acute renal failure?

20 minutes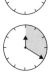

Question four: What are the possible nursing interventions and medical treatment that Mrs Fairhead will require?

25 minutes

Time allowance: **60 minutes**

Answer to question one:
Define the term acute renal failure.

Acute renal failure (ARF) occurs suddenly and there is an almost complete loss of renal function characterised by an accumulation of nitrogenous waste products in the circulating blood that is not caused by extra-renal factors and is reversible (Paradisco, 1999). Renal originates from the Latin word ren, meaning kidney. Nepr is from Greek word nephros and also means kidney. In this instance, renal, appertaining to the kidney is used appropriately here (Hutton, 1993).

Answer to question two:
What are the possible causes of acute renal failure?

Any one of the following can cause acute renal failure:

1. In pre-renal ARF the prolonged reduction of blood flow (e.g. hypovolaemia due to blood loss or severe burns and dehydration, aortic stenosis, renal artery disease) to the kidneys cause them to fail to work especially the ability to rid the body of wastes.
2. In renal ARF there is damage to the renal parenchyma due to glomerulonephritis, acute tubular necrosis, diabetic nephropathy, pyelonephritis and toxic drugs. In the case of Mrs Fairhead acute renal failure is a result of an acute haemolytic transfusion reaction.
3. Post-renal ARF is caused by an obstruction to urine outflow due to renal stones, bilateral ureteric stricture, prostatic hypertrophy and external tumours that compress the ureters.

Answer to question three:
What are the pathophysiological manifestations of acute renal failure?

The pathophysiological manifestations of ARF can be divided into three distinctive phases (Frizzell, 2001) related to the functions of the kidneys.

1. The acute onset phase – the period from the acute episode to the onset of oliguria and anuria. This oliguria-anuria period usually lasts for between 1 and 2 weeks, during which there is a reduction of urinary output of less than 400 ml per day to no urinary output. Obviously, the longer duration means that the prognosis is poor. This is the phase in which toxins accumulate. The rising blood urea nitrogen (BUN) and creatinine measure this. The patient will experience metabolic acidosis when there is a higher than normal accumulation of acids.

2. Early diuretic phase – this signifies that the kidneys are recovering and as such the urinary output will rise gradually and the BUN will fall. Late diuretic and recovery phase – the period in which the BUN falls to within the normal range.

3. Convalescent phase – the period in which the BUN is stable and daily urine output is normal and the patient resumes normal activity.

Answer to question four:
What are the possible nursing interventions and medical treatment that Mrs Fairhead will require?

Mrs Fairhead will be very anxious and distressed about her illness and her loss of independence. Consequently, Mrs Fairhead should be assessed according to her individualised and holistic needs (Walsh, 1997) so that an individualised care plan can be formulated. Mrs Fairhead should be given adequate information, support and reassurance so that her anxiety can be allayed. Any treatment and procedures carried out should be explained beforehand to gain trust and cooperation from her.

Mrs Fairhead's sons should be kept informed and updated on their mother's condition.

The assessment of Mrs Fairhead's electrolytes, fluid intake and output, acids and bases can provide an indication of whether her kidneys are recovering.

The nurse must maintain a strict intake and output record. The intake of fluids is normally determined by the previous day's output plus insensible loss due to sweating, breathing and elimination of faeces. Insensible loss varies according to the size of the patient and also if the patient is suffering from a pyrexia. The correct assessment of fluid intake ensures that only losses are replaced as overloading of fluids may cause pulmonary oedema.

As a result of the high level of urea in the blood there is a need to reduce the amount of protein intake between 14 and 20 grams per day (Dudek, 2001). In order to prevent catabolism (breakdown of cells and potassium is released) sufficient amount of fat and carbohydrate are introduced into the diet.

Due to the high level of potassium, Mrs Fairhead should avoid foods rich in potassium such as bananas, cocoa and citrus fruits. Iron exchange resins (Calcium Resonium) can also be given to withdraw potassium from the gastrointestinal tract. Sometimes insulin can be given with glucose to make the cells more permeable to potassium. When potassium enters the cells serum potassium should be lowered and likelihood of any cardiac arrhythmias can be curtailed. Resting Mrs Fairhead can also reduce catabolism, however, due to reduced mobility, Mrs Fairhead must be assessed for any risks of pressure ulcers.

There are a few complications associated with ARF that the nurse must be made aware of. These include hyperkalaemia (high serum potassium level), cardiac arrhythmias, convulsions and eventually coma. Therefore, the nurse must observe for any clinical symptoms associated with potassium intoxication, which include muscle weakness, changes in respiration, parasthesia in the limbs and around the mouth, hypotension and cardiac arrhythmias that may precipitate a cardiac arrest.

Early detection of any cardiac rhythms is essential, therefore Mrs Fairhead's cardiac status should be monitored and any cardiac abnormalities must be corrected immediately by intravenous medications.

The nurse must observe any early signs of muscular twitching that precipitate a convulsion. Anticonvulsive drugs may be prescribed to control or prevent any further seizures.

If Mrs Fairhead's condition does not improve then peritoneal or haemodialysis can be commenced to maintain the fluid and electrolyte balance.

Client profiles in nursing: adult & the elderly 2

References

Dudek, S.G. (2001) Nutrition Essentials for Nursing Practice. (4th ed.). New York: Lippincott.

Frizzell, J.P. (2001) Handbook of Pathophysiology: Causes, Signs and Symptoms, Disease Management. Pennsylvania: Springhouse Corporation.

Hutton, A.R. (1993) An Introduction to Medical Terminology: A Self-Teaching Package. London: Churchill Livingstone.

Paradisco, C. (1999) Lippincott's Review Series: The Ideal Study Aid. Here's Why…. Pathophysiology. (2nd ed.). New York: Lippincott.

Walsh, M. (1997) Watson's Clinical Nursing & Related Science. (5th ed.). London: Bailliere Tindall.

Further reading

Abrams, A.C. (2001) Clinical Drug Therapy: Rationales for Nursing Practice. New York: Lippincott.

Unresolved grief in the elderly

Chris Buswell

Mrs Lillian Hartnell is a 78-year-old widow. Her husband, Ian, a retired television producer, died 7 years ago. They had one child, Mary, who died when she was 7 months old. Mrs Hartnell's only living relative is her nephew, Graham. For the last 6 months Mrs Hartnell has lived in a nursing home as she has dementia. Before then she was looked after in her home by privately funded carers. Her nephew arranged for her to move from her house to a nursing home near to his village. Although Mrs Hartnell is able to recall events in her past, she suffers from forgetfulness and short term memory loss. She has no other health care problems, other than an inability to initiate any self care. When prompted and with minimal assistance she can wash and dress herself, feed herself and mobilise around the nursing home, although at times she will wander into other people's rooms.

'Hello Mrs Hartnell,' said Abigail as she entered Mrs Hartnell's room. 'I've come to tidy your cupboard out whilst I've got a spare few minutes. Is that okay?'

'Yes dear, have you seen Mary? Only she isn't in her cot.' 'No Mrs Hartnell you're in a nursing home and I'm Abigail, your carer for this morning.'

Abigail started tidying Mrs Hartnell's cupboard by taking down a shoe box. 'I'll take these shoes out of their box so you can get the use of them.' When she opened the box Abigail was surprised to find a tiny pair of baby shoes and some old, musty photographs of a baby. She laid them on the bed. As Mrs Hartnell saw them she started to rock in her chair and cry. 'Oh Mary, oh Mary,' she wailed.

Abigail walked over to Mrs Hartnell and put a comforting arm around her. 'It's all right to cry, but whatever is the matter?' she asked.

Between sobs Mrs Hartnell kept repeating, 'Mary, Mary.'

'Was this your baby Mrs Hartnell?' asked Abigail gently.

Mrs Hartnell nodded her head and hugged Abigail tightly. 'Oh how I miss her. Taken away from me so suddenly. Ian and I loved her so much and then one day she was gone. He never wanted to talk about her. Oh Mary,' screamed Mrs Hartnell as she began to cry again.

Question one: Discuss unresolved grief and how this might affect people, like Mrs Hartnell, in later life.

25 minutes

Question two: Describe ways in which the nursing and care staff might help Mrs Hartnell resolve and come to terms with her past losses.

20 minutes

Time allowance: **45 minutes**

Answer to question one:
Discuss unresolved grief and how this might affect people, like Mrs Hartnell, in later life.

As people age others may assume that they have coped with any past bereavements and losses, accepted them and moved on (Heath & Schofield, 1999; Tschudin, 1999). However this is not always the case. As can be seen in the case study, unresolved grief may resurface years later. Elderly people, with more free time and more thinking time may review their life and feel a sense of loss at past events, people or objects, rather than feelings of a sense of worth and having lived a full and enjoyable life. As with any age group, elderly people may need the assistance of skilful and empathic care staff to help them accept and learn to live with their loss.

Earlier losses faced by the elderly may be compounded as they have to deal with other losses such as employment, status, reduced income, death of loved ones, friends or family, independence, failing health and, like Mrs Hartnell, a change of surroundings and loss of a family home (Eliopoulos, 1993; Heath & Schofield, 1999; Hicks, 2000; Tschudin, 1999).

Some people think that the death of a child is the most difficult form of grief an older person can face (Heath & Schofield, 1999). Perhaps more so for someone like Mrs Hartnell who may feel that Mary had no chance to live her life and was suddenly and cruelly taken from her and her husband. Mr and Mrs Hartnell may have lived in an age when emotions and feelings were suppressed and a stoical 'get on with life' attitude may have been evident. Not being able to talk through her grief with her husband may have been very difficult for Mrs Hartnell.

People, like Mrs Hartnell, in nursing homes away from long term friends and apart from their family may suffer detrimentally and can feel little attachment to other residents and staff (Hicks, 2000). This may increase feelings of loneliness, grief and loss. An increase in dependency may increase feelings of loneliness and grief (Gould, 1992; Hicks, 2000).

Grief may manifest itself as signs of extreme stress such as decreased attentiveness and alertness, insomnia, confusion, disorientation and behavioural problems. Elderly people face the risk of such reactions to grief being inappropriately diagnosed as dementia (Hegge & Fischer, 2000).

Answer to question two:
Describe ways in which the nursing and care staff might help Mrs Hartnell resolve and come to terms with her past losses.

A common theme throughout the literature which discusses bereavement and loss is that the grieving individual needs to reach a state of peace to achieve a level of acceptance and resolution but, sadly, not all individuals do (Cutcliffe, 1998). Nurses and care assistants have a duty of care to their patients to assist them in reaching such resolution. Staff in residential and nursing homes who build more meaningful and deeper relationships with their patients are in an ideal position to help them to reach an acceptance of their losses through the use of counselling and inter-personal skills.

Such skills include active listening (Heath & Schofield, 1999; Hicks, 2000; Manthei, 1997; McMahon & Isaacs, 1997; Tschudin, 1999), warmth (Tschudin, 1999), genuineness (Bayne, Nicolson & Horton, 1998; Tschudin, 1999) and empathy (Bayne, Nicolson & Horton, 1998; Heath & Schofield, 1999; Manthei, 1997; Tschudin, 1999). For an explanation of these terms please refer to Volume One: Case Five; Mrs Dorothy Bell (Buswell, 2001).

Abigail, the carer, has initiated the grieving process for Mrs Hartnell by acknowledging that it is good to cry and allowing Mrs Hartnell to hug her (McMahon & Isaacs, 1997).

Counselling performed by staff need not be formal counselling in the true sense, but structured periods of what may seem to Mrs Hartnell to be purely conversations. Nursing and care staff can help Mrs Hartnell talk about her feelings surrounding Mary and Mr Hartnell. Staff may also want to discuss other losses that Mrs Hartnell has suffered such as the loss of her home.

Mrs Hartnell may benefit from reminiscence therapy (Bruce, Hodgson & Schweitzer, 1999) to help her value her life and look back at fond memories. Staff could assist her to display the photographs of Mary, or to talk about memories such as bathing or feeding Mary. Staff with their own children could talk over how they care for their baby compared with how it was in Mrs Hartnell's day. A display of photographs could include some of her husband.

Staff could discuss with Mrs Hartnell the positive effects of moving home. Talking about visits from Mrs Hartnell's nephew could reinforce the positive aspects of the move and increase her interaction with the staff. Discussion with Mrs Hartnell's nephew about the grief still felt by Mrs Hartnell might make him and his family more involved in her care. Nursing staff could suggest regular visits from his family to help reduce Mrs Hartnell's feelings of loneliness, as could visits from volunteers and other patients (Hegge & Fischer, 2000; Hicks, 2000).

Nurses and care staff in nursing and residential homes are ideally placed to facilitate interaction between patients in an attempt to reduce their feelings of loneliness (Hicks, 2000).

References

Bayne, R., Nicolson, P., Horton, I. (Eds) (1998) Counselling and Communication Skills for Medical and Health Practitioners. Leicester: The British Psychological Society.

Bruce, E., Hodgson, S., Schweitzer, P. (1999) Reminiscing With People With Dementia. London: Age Exchange.

Buswell, C. (2001) Case five: Miss D. Bell: Alzheimer's disease: validation therapy: reality orientation: communication. In: Simpson, P., Okubadejo, T. (Eds). Client Profiles in Nursing: Adult and the Elderly. London: Greenwich Medical Media, pp 31–36.

Cutcliffe, J.R. (1998) Hope, counselling and complicated bereavement reactions. Journal of Advanced Nursing 28(4): 754–761.

Eliopoulos, C. (1993) Gerontological Nursing. (3rd ed.). Philadelphia: J.B. Lippincott Company.

Gould, M. (1992) Nursing home elderly: social-environmental factors. Journal of Gerontological Nursing 18(8): 13–20.

Heath, H., Schofield, I. (Ed.) (1999) Healthy Ageing: Nursing Older People. London: Mosby.

Hegge, M., Fischer, C. (2000) Grief responses of senior and elderly widows. Journal of Gerontological Nursing 26(2): 35–43.

Hicks, T.J. (2000) What is your life like now? Loneliness and elderly individuals residing in nursing homes. Journal of Gerontological Nursing 26(8): 15–19.

Manthei, R. (1997) Counselling: The Skills of Finding Solutions to Problems. London: Routledge.

McMahon, C., Isaacs, R. (Eds) (1997) Care of the Older Person. Oxford: Blackwell Science.

Tschudin, V. (Ed.) (1999) Counselling and Older People. London: Age Concern.

Caring

Penny Tremayne

Mildred Chapman is a 78-year-old widow who is admitted to a general medical ward as a 'social problem' following an increasing number of falls at home. Mrs Chapman lives alone in a three bedroom detached house on the outskirts of a town. She has two grown up children. Her son Doug lives in a bordering county with his wife and son; he is rarely in contact with his mother. Mrs Chapman's daughter Angela visits every Sunday afternoon with her husband to take her mother out for lunch.

Since the death of her husband 8 years ago, Mrs Chapman has immersed herself into church activities. She is also a volunteer for a charity shop in town. She has many close friends who live locally and who call to see her throughout the week.

Ill health has plagued Mrs Chapman over the past 5 years. She has had an aortic valve replacement and takes medications for non-insulin dependant diabetes, hypertension and osteoporosis. Last year Mrs Chapman slipped on some ice and fractured her right wrist. Just 4 months ago she fractured her right tibia after tripping down a step. Even with the use of a walking stick Mrs Chapman's falls are becoming more frequent. Consequently her confidence is much reduced and she is struggling to maintain her home. She eats irregularly and often relies on friends and neighbours for her shopping and meals. More recently she has become increasingly forgetful and at times slightly confused. She has confined herself to living downstairs and her brother-in-law is currently converting a room downstairs into a shower room.

On admission Mrs Chapman has bruises and grazes to her limbs as well as cuts and grazes to her face.

After 2 days in hospital, Mrs Chapman's daughter visits and is alarmed to find her mother in the same nightdress. Mrs Chapman indicated that she had not been offered a wash since admission. Her daughter makes a verbal complaint to the ward manager about the care her mother has been receiving.

Question one: How could nurses have initially demonstrated that they 'care' for Mrs Chapman?

15 minutes

Question two: Discuss the essential care that Mrs Chapman will require in relation to health care policy.

20 minutes

Question three: Explain how the ward manager should handle the complaint.

15 minutes

Time allowance: **50 minutes**

Client profiles in nursing: adult & the elderly 2

Answer to question one:
How could nurses have initially demonstrated that they 'care' for Mrs Chapman?

Mrs Chapman should be welcomed to the ward. To promote comfort she should have the option to rest on either a bed with an appropriate mattress or chair with pressure relieving cushion, whichever she prefers.

To enhance Mrs Chapman's understanding of what is going on, the nurse should explain who he/she is, and his/her actions and ensure that Mrs Chapman informally consents to these. Aware that Mrs Chapman may be tired and in need of rest, she should be allowed to indicate what she would prefer to do. Person-centred care and services are important to Mrs Chapman as this can facilitate an individualised approach to her care (Department of Health, 2001a).

The call bell system should be explained and provided within easy and safe reach so that she has the ability other than verbal to communicate her needs. Effective communication is a key factor in making Mrs Chapman feel cared for; this can be done verbally or non verbally. When verbally communicating an appropriate tone, pace and volume of voice should always be adopted. A question such as 'what can we do to make you feel more comfortable' can be used to facilitate the identification of Mrs Chapman's initial needs. Of equal importance is the role of being an active listener and responding appropriately to what Mrs Chapman is communicating (Department of Health, 2001a). The nurse should be aware of the impact of their non-verbal communication. A smile, the use of touch, acting in a professional, competent, confident manner can also communicate caring to Mrs Chapman.

Mrs Chapman could be introduced to key areas such as toilets, bathroom, telephone points and her bed and living space identified so she can begin to familiarise herself with the new surroundings and the layout of the ward. Mrs Chapman should be allowed the choice as to whether she wishes to wear her own clothes and to have her personal effects at her bedside (Department of Health, 2001a). Continuous repetition of information may be necessary as Mrs Chapman is confused and forgetful.

Mrs Chapman may feel thirsty or hungry so she should be offered, provided and assisted with appropriate drinks and diet.

Answer to question two:
Discuss the essential care that Mrs Chapman will require in relation to health care policy.

A single assessment process which bridges both health and social care should include consideration of the following elements: the user perspective, clinical background, disease prevention, personal care and physical well being, senses, mental health, relationships, safety, immediate environment and resources (Department of Health, 2001a). This should be conducted as soon as possible so an individualised care plan can be formulated which takes into account the acute care, and the scope of rehabilitation which will finally inform the discharge process of Mrs Chapman.

Good management of care will require attention according to the Department of Health (2001a) to the following: maintaining fluid balance, pain management, pressure sore risk management, acute confusion, falls and immobility, nutritional status and risk management, cognitive impairment, rehabilitation potential, depression, infection control, medicines management, social circumstances, family and other carer's needs, how and where to access other specialist services and end of life care. Mrs Chapman will require active rehabilitation, amongst which her falls and mental health needs will be individually addressed. Nationally, the basic or rather fundamental aspects of care that is delivered to patients like Mrs Chapman is variable. The Department of Health (2001b) in a bid to bridge the gap between the best and the rest introduced clinical practice benchmarking. This quality initiative can be defined as '... a process through which best practice is identified and continuous improvement pursued through comparison and sharing' (Department of Health, 1999, 49).

The fundamental aspects of care that Mrs Chapman will require are:

- Personal and oral hygiene
- Privacy and dignity
- Pressure ulcer prevention
- Continence and bladder and bowel care
- Food and nutrition
- Possible safety of people with mental illness (occasional confusion).

Department of Health (2001b)

Answer to question three:
Explain how the ward manager should handle the complaint.

- Listen and try to understand instead of deflecting the blame. The ward manager should make it clear that the complaint is being taken seriously and that the ward team and the unit manager will be involved
- Offer to take Mrs Chapman's daughter to a side room or an office
- Be open and honest and reassure Mrs Chapman's daughter that the complaint will not compromise the care her mother is receiving
- Apologise.

These actions can have a profound effect on the way the complaint progresses. It is integral that good records are maintained and that a record of a complaint such as this one is made and local policy/protocol applied.

References

Department of Health (1999) Making a Difference: Strengthening the Nursing, Midwifery and Health Visiting Contribution to Health and Healthcare. London: The Stationery Office.

Department of Health (2001a) Modern Standards and Service Models: National Service Framework for Older People. London: The Stationery Office.

Department of Health (2001b) Essence of Care: Patient-focused Benchmarking for Health Care Practitioners. London: The Stationery Office.

Further reading

Department of Health (1991) The Patient's Charter. London: HMSO.

Department of Health (1996) The NHS Complaints Procedure. London: The Stationery Office.

Gunn, C. (2001) A Practical Guide to Complaints Handling: In the Context of Clinical Governance. London: Churchill Livingstone.

National Health Service Executive (1996) Complaints ... Acting ... Improving: Guidance on implementation of the NHS Complaints Procedure. London: The Stationery Office.

Rowbotham, M. (2001) How to handle complaints. Nursing Times 97(30): 25–28.

United Kingdom Central Council for Nursing, Midwifery and Health Visiting (UKCC) (1998) Complaints About Professional Conduct. (2nd ed.). London: UKCC.

Tuberculosis

Maggie Chappell

Melissa Walker is a 35-year-old housewife. She lives in a 3 bedroom maisonette with her husband and their two daughters in a rural village. Duncan, her husband, has been unemployed for about a year. The girls, Jenny aged 9 years and Sarah aged 6 years both attend the local primary school. Both Melissa and Duncan have been born and brought up in the same village and do not like to travel abroad, preferring local holidays.

Melissa looks after Emily, her friend's 2-year-old daughter, for several hours every day while her mother goes to work. She has 2 other primary school children to look after at the end of the school day for about an hour. She is not registered as a child minder but does it as a favour for friends.

Melissa smoked 10 cigarettes a day until 6 months ago when she gave up completely because she was unwell. Her husband still smokes. She rarely drinks alcohol and does not take any regular medication except the oral contraceptive pill. She has had all the recommended vaccinations at each stage of her life, including the Bacille Calmette-Guerin (BCG) vaccine against tuberculosis (TB) at the age of 14 years.

Melissa has been unwell for at least 12 months. She has had persistent problems with her chest. She has had five courses of antibiotics and been given inhalers to help with her productive cough and feelings of chest tightness and wheeze. She has lost weight; initially the weight loss was slow but over the last 6 weeks she has lost 10 kg. She has had frequent night sweats and is having to get up in the night to wash and change her clothes and sometimes the sheets. She feels exhausted and is becoming low in mood.

Melissa has just been admitted to hospital. She came to the Accident and Emergency department after coughing up about half a cupful of fresh blood. A provisional diagnosis of pulmonary TB was made and she was hospitalised.

Question one: What is tuberculosis?

Question two: Describe how it is transmitted

Question three: List the investigations th confirm the disease.

Question four: Describe the treatment for tuberculosis and consider the potential side effects that Melissa should be warned about.

30 minutes

Time allowance: **60 minutes**

Answer to question one:
What is tuberculosis?

Tuberculosis is the disease caused by infection with *Mycobacterium tuberculosis* or, *M. bovis* or *M. africanum* (Marchant, 1998). Although any organ in the body may be affected, it is most commonly found in the lungs. The bacillus is a very slow growing organism so the onset of symptoms is usually insidious and symptoms are often non-specific in nature.

Answer to question two:
Describe how it is transmitted.

Tuberculosis is transmitted from person to person when someone who has pulmonary tuberculosis disease coughs and mycobacteria are expelled in the droplets of sputum. These can then be inhaled by other people. It generally takes close and prolonged contact for transmission to occur. Typically, less than 10% of contacts followed up during contact tracing show any evidence of infection (Mackay, 1993). Tuberculosis is not infectious in any site other than the lungs unless exudate from the area is aerosolised, for example if irrigation of a tuberculous lesion is performed.

The initial infection with *M. tuberculosis* is called primary tuberculosis. It is usually symptomless. Some individuals may have brief 'flu-like' symptoms some weeks after their exposure to an infectious case of tuberculosis. These usually resolve without treatment. In some 20% of people who have had primary tuberculosis the mycobacteria remain in a dormant form (Smales, 1999). Dormant tuberculosis infection leaves that individual with the life-long potential for the mycobacteria to re-activate and make that person ill with tuberculosis disease. That person will not know they have dormant tuberculosis infection. The mycobacteria are not visible on X-ray, they do not cause any symptoms and are not transmissible to others.

Any significant pressure on the body's immune system may allow the re-activation of dormant tuberculosis infection. The onset of another illness, a period of severe stress, the use of certain immuno-suppressive drugs are examples of such triggers. The mycobacteria then start to multiply and eventually to cause symptoms. It is usually only after the symptoms have been present for several months that there are sufficient numbers of mycobacteria in the sputum for the patient to be infectious.

Answer to question three:
List the investigations that can be carried out to confirm the disease.

History

The diagnosis is often delayed because of the non-specific nature of the symptoms of tuberculosis and the slow insidious onset of symptoms. The symptoms will vary according to the site(s) of infection but a careful history of the illness is vital. If the site of infection is in a joint there will be local pain and swelling and in the renal tract there will be signs associated with urinary tract infection. Regardless of the site, most patients will experience fatigue and some degree of weight loss as the body tries to protect itself from this potentially overwhelming disease. Many patients will also complain of night sweats which can be drenching. These are because of typical evening low-grade pyrexias which resolve during the night, accompanied by profuse sweating.

Patients with pulmonary tuberculosis will usually experience a cough, initially dry but gradually becoming more productive of sputum (Cowle, 1995). They may have some chest pain or discomfort and they may have haemoptysis. Some have such paroxysms of coughing that they vomit. They may see their General Practitioner (GP) and be given antibiotics but any relief resulting from them will be short lived.

X-ray

Pulmonary tuberculosis often presents with typical chest X-ray changes making the diagnosis easier.

Suspicion of tuberculosis in any part of the body should trigger a request for a chest X-ray because the initial primary infection with tuberculosis can leave a small calcified 'scar' on the lung which may also be a diagnostic aid. X-rays of the affected part of the body may be helpful also.

Microbiology

The acquisition of samples of sputum, urine or tissue is of huge importance in the diagnosis and confirmation of tuberculosis (Joint Tuberculosis Committee, 2000). Laboratories need to be requested to do specific tests for *M. tuberculosis*, as they are not routinely performed. The specimen is stained and examined under the microscope. The presence of mycobacteria can be very helpful in making the diagnosis. Unfortunately, culture confirmation of the species of mycobacterium takes up to 8 weeks so treatment must be initiated before confirmation is made. The other essential part microbiology plays is the establishment of the sensitivities of the organism cultured to the specific antibiotics used to treat tuberculosis. As drug-resistance becomes more of a problem, world-wide, it is vital to treat patients appropriately.

If a patient is unable to produce sputum, bronchoscopy may be considered in order to obtain specimens. In cases of suspected non-pulmonary tuberculosis, aspiration or surgical biopsy will enable the acquisition of specimens which must not be put in formalin as that kills organisms.

Tuberculin testing

This is a procedure carried out by appropriately trained nurses who can also interpret the results. An amount of Purified Protein Derivative of *M. tuberculosis* is injected intradermally on the patient's forearm. This initiates a response and the test is regarded as positive if 2–4 days after injection, there is a reaction consisting of a raised area of inflammatory oedema, not less than 5 mm in diameter, with surrounding erythema. Unfortunately the test is not specific to *M. tuberculosis* but will react to the presence of other mycobacteria (there are more than 80 in the environment). The test has to be interpreted carefully, taking into account the patient's immune status. Any depression of the immune system's ability to react to the stimulus of a tuberculin test will result in a false negative reaction. This can be caused by the disease process of tuberculosis itself.

Answer to question four:

Describe the treatment for tuberculosis and consider the potential side effects that Melissa should be warned about.

Patients are given a combination of specific antibiotics for a period of at least 6 months. There are slight variations around the world but generally they are given three or four ('triple' or 'quadruple' therapy). After 2 months of this regimen, assuming they are making good progress and they have fully sensitive organisms, they are changed to a regimen of only two drugs (Mitchson, 2000). All of the drugs are potentially toxic. Many patients complain of nausea, fatigue and small joint pains in the first couple of weeks of treatment. The treatment should be taken in a single dose on an empty stomach. After the first 2 weeks of treatment the patient is considered non-infectious.

There are different tablet preparations available containing two or three of the anti-tuberculous drugs. Many of the drugs and combinations have names beginning with 'Rif' so dispensing errors are a risk.

Rifampicin

This is given for the full 6 months of treatment. It stains all body fluids red or orange so Melissa will notice the colour of her urine and faeces changes. It will even stain soft contact lenses. It interferes with the action of some other drugs including the oral contraceptive pill so Melissa will need advice on an alternative method of contraception. It rarely causes a hepatitis-type reaction (Thong-Ngam Kullavanijaya 2002) which is potentially very serious so Melissa needs to be warned to stop her treatment if she develops this. Early signs are nausea, fatigue and itchy skin. The onset of jaundice means she must stop treatment and seek medical advice urgently. She will have regular blood tests to monitor for this reaction.

Isoniazid

This is given for the full 6 months of treatment. It may give rise to a peripheral neuropathy so Melissa should be warned to notice and report tingling or pins and needles in her hands and toes. Taking Pyridoxine daily helps to prevent this side effect.

This drug can also cause a hepatitis-type reaction as above.

Pyrazinamide

This is discontinued after the first 2 months of treatment. It can cause hepatic toxicity as above.

Ethambutol

This is discontinued after the first 2 months of treatment. It can cause problems with vision so Melissa should be warned to stop taking this drug and seek

Client profiles in nursing: adult & the elderly 2

medical attention if she notices any deterioration in her visual acuity or colour blindness for green.

References

Cowle, R. (1995) TB: cure, care and control. Nursing Times 91(38): 29–30.

Joint Tuberculosis Committee of the British Thoracic Society (2000) Control and prevention of tuberculosis in the United Kingdom: code of practice. Thorax Journal 55: 887–901.

Mackay, L. (1993) Evaluation is the key to success: a nurse-led tuberculosis contact-tracing service. Professional Nurse 9(3): 176–180.

Marchant, N. (1998) Tuberculosis: London. Office of Health Economics.

Mitchson, D. (2000) Role of individual drugs in the chemotherapy of tuberculosis. International Journal of Tuberculosis and Lung Disease 4(9): 796–806.

Smales, C. (1999) Return of the silent killer. Nursing Times 95(35): 59.

Thong-Ngam, D., Kullavanijaya, P. (2002) Antituberculous-drug-induced hepatotoxicity. International Journal of Gastroenterology 6(1): 18–21.

Further reading

Bhatti, N., Law, M.R. et al (1995) Increasing incidence of tuberculosis in England and Wales: a study of the likely causes. British Medical Journal 310: 967–969.

Rose, A.M.C., Watson, J.M. et al (2001) Tuberculosis at the end of the 20th century in England and Wales: results of a national survey in 1998. Thorax Journal 56: 173–179.

Useful websites

British Thoracic Society: www.brit-thoracic.org.uk
World Health Organization: www.who.ch/gtb

Useful address

British Thoracic Society
17 Doughty Street
London
WC1N 2PL

Sexuality and the ageing process

Chris Buswell

'I feel so alive nurse, I never thought I'd feel like this again, not at my age, 76 next week in fact,' confided Catherine to Malcolm. 'It's as if I've been reborn, with new experiences and fresh hopes and dreams. When I first came to this home I didn't dream I'd find someone else. After Phillip died I was so low. I didn't want to do anything, or want to know anybody. I even turned my back on my own children. I'm sure that must have upset them. Especially when they came to visit me several weeks later and found me in such a state. I hadn't eaten for days, I hadn't bothered to wash or change my clothes. My house was in such a mess. But now they can see the change in me, and I feel so close to them and my grandchildren. I had a superb dinner with them last week and for the first time I was so glad to come back to the nursing home. I even heard myself calling it my home to the children. It's strange to think that when I first came here I did so reluctantly. My children thought I couldn't care for myself and needed care so arranged for me to come into the local home, into the residential wing. At first I was so angry with them, and with everyone really. I was rather rude to everybody and quite snappy. One patient persevered with me, coming into my room for chats, delivering the daily newspaper and mail. We got talking and soon discovered that we had so much in common. After a few months we got close, kissing and cuddling. It was a closeness neither of us imagined we'd experience again after our lifelong partners died. It wasn't long before we found ourselves in bed. Mind you we were a bit embarrassed at first. We'd always lock the door in case a member of staff came into the room. It was fun going into each others' rooms though. It made me feel like a naughty teenager. That is part of the excitement. Another exciting part of our relationship is finding new ways of love making that don't cause any problems with my arthritis. In a way that makes it more intimate and tender. There's no rush to have sex since we've got all day. We've no pressures or worries. Sometimes we just lie in bed cuddling without a care in the world. I'm glad you understand nurse and it's nice to talk about how I feel towards Elizabeth.'

Question one: Describe the physical changes that can affect sexual intercourse that elderly women may experience as they age.

30 minutes

Question two: Discuss lesbianism in the elderly.

30 minutes

Time allowance: **60 minutes**

Answer to question one:
Describe the physical changes that can affect sexual intercourse that elderly women may experience as they age.

As people age there are many natural changes that will affect them physically. Such natural changes may affect women of any sexual orientation.

As women age there may be a decrease in sexual responsiveness (Eliopoulos, 1993; Heath & Schofield, 1999; Russell, 1998), although some older women gain a new interest in sex, perhaps because they no longer have to fear pregnancy or have no commitments such as children or careers, or have more privacy and time (Drench & Losee, 1996; Eliopoulos, 1993; Gibson, 1997b; Parke, 1991). However Tortora & Grabowski (1996) argue that there is no change in libido due to the continued production of adrenal adrogens. Other authors describe no change in sexual desire (Grigg, 1999).

Older women may experience pain or discomfort during intercourse (dyspareunia) due to vaginal dryness caused by a decreased level of oestrogen (Eliopoulos, 1993; Gibson, 1997b; Grigg, 1999; Heath & Schofield, 1999; McMahon & Isaacs, 1997; Parke, 1991; Russell, 1998; Tortora & Grabowski, 1996) and atrophy of the vaginal and distal urethral epithelium (Heath, 2000). These factors also cause a change in the pH balance (Heath, 2000). Vaginal dryness can be overcome by applying a lubricating solution before or during sexual intercourse (Gibson, 1997b; Russell, 1998). Other causes of dyspareunia may be decreased distensibility and thinning of the vaginal walls (Eliopoulos, 1993; Heath, 1999; Heath & Schofield, 1999).

Elderly women may experience a reduction in the frequency of orgasm (Eliopoulos, 1993; Russell, 1998) or find that orgasm takes longer to achieve and the sensation of orgasm is reduced (Heath, 1999), women who have regular sexual intercourse being able to achieve orgasm (Grigg, 1999; Parke, 1991). Grigg (1999) and Heath (1999) describe orgasms as being beneficial to urinary continence and maintaining muscle tone. Some elderly women may experience uterine spasm during orgasm (Parke, 1991).

As women age the vagina becomes narrower (Eliopoulos, 1993; Heath & Schofield, 1999; McMahon & Isaacs, 1997; Tortora & Grabowski, 1996) and the clitoris decreases in size (McMahon & Isaacs, 1997; Tortora & Grabowski, 1996), some elderly women may find clitoral stimulation painful (Parke, 1991). During the excitement phase of the sexual response cycle the labia majora does not separate, flatten or elevate (Eliopoulos, 1993; Heath & Schofield, 1999), there are reduced reactions to the labia minora (Eliopoulos, 1993; Heath & Schofield, 1999), and the Bartholin's glands secrete less mucus (Eliopoulos, 1993; Heath & Schofield, 1999). Sexual plateau is of a reduced intensity (Eliopoulos, 1993; Heath & Schofield, 1999) and during orgasm there are the same vaginal contractions experienced by younger women but the duration is shorter (Eliopoulos, 1993; Grigg, 1999; Heath & Schofield, 1999).

Breasts become more pendulous (Heath, 2000) and pubic hair thins and becomes more scanty (Heath, 2000). The labia majora and minora become thinner, may flatten and hangs in folds (Heath, 2000).

Older women can still experience the same common factors as younger women that can inhibit fulfilling sexual intercourse. Such factors include anxiety, low self esteem, stress and depression, an unsuitable environment with lack of privacy, distractions or noise and the negative attitude of carers (Cole, 2001; Heath, 1999; McMahon & Isaacs, 1997; Parke, 1991).

Older women, like Catherine, may suffer from chronic medical conditions and painful or debilitating illnesses that may make sexual intercourse painful or uncomfortable (Cole, 2001; Heath, 1999; Irwin, 2000; Le Gallez, 1998; Parke, 1991). Conditions such as arthritis may make certain sexual positions uncomfortable or painful (Heath, 1999; Le Gallez, 1998; Parke, 1991). Patients may find it beneficial to seek advice and counselling regarding alternative sexual techniques or positions (Gibson, 1997b; Le Gallez, 1998; McMahon & Isaacs, 1997; Parke, 1991). Nurses and care assistants must take such requests seriously, without embarrassment, and be prepared to refer patients to appropriate outside professional agencies.

Elderly patients may have polypharmacy and be suffering side effects of medications. Certain drugs such as antihypertensives, antidepressants, diuretics, antipsychotics and anticholinergics may cause sexual problems (Heath, 1999; Heath, 2000; Irwin, 2000; Parke, 1991; Russell, 1998). For example some medications may cause vaginal candida (Drench & Losee, 1996) others, like Levodopa may cause excessive and inappropriate sexual behaviour (Parke, 1991), whilst antihistamines decrease vaginal lubrication (Russell, 1998).

Answer to question two:
Discuss lesbianism in the elderly.

Stereotypical perceptions of the elderly are that they are sexless and sexually inactive (Brogan, 1996; Gibson, 1997a; Heath & Schofield, 1999; Heath & White, 2001; Parke, 1991; Russell, 1998; Tschudin, 2000). The media portray the elderly with images and advertisements of laxatives, insurance and thermal underwear (Ford, 1998) indulging in pastimes such as knitting and bingo (Gibson, 1997a). However the sexual needs and sexuality of the elderly are complex, sensitive and often covert (Grigg, 2000; Heath & Schofield, 1999). Elderly sex is still seen as the greatest taboo subject in today's society (Heath, 2000; Thomas, 1999). The older lesbian, such as Catherine, may be faced with prejudiced views and stereotypical attitudes (McMahon & Isaacs, 1997) and her health and social needs ignored because health care professionals lack adequate information and sensitivity to her needs (Deevey, 1990; Heath & Schofield, 1999). Deevey (1990) considers that elderly lesbians are in a triple minority because of their age, sexual orientation and gender. Elderly women are seen as less attractive and sexually ineligible at a younger age than elderly men (Grigg, 1999). Deevey (1990) further describes the prejudiced views and myths stereotypical towards elderly lesbians as unhappy, childless, man looking women. In her study of 78 lesbians aged between 50–82 Deevey (1990) discovered that one third, like Catherine, had had children and forty percent had in fact been married. Of the same sample 80% of the women were happy with their own aging although only nine percent had revealed their true sexuality to others.

Elderly women were brought up not to discuss the taboo subject of sex, which was seen as vulgar and an act for married women for procreational purposes (Eliopoulos, 1993; Gibson, 1997b; Parke, 1991; Russell, 1998). Fortunately such stigmas and prejudices are changing and individuality and sexual preferences are now more widely accepted (Deevey, 1990; Gibson, 1997a). However nurses and carers may still hear older lesbians describe feelings of guilt and anxiety. Some gay women may feel embarrassed or uneasy with their sexuality and may lead a secretive life, remain isolated, be fearful or anxious, and may be uncomfortable with disclosure (Deevey, 1990; McMahon & Isaacs, 1997).

Homosexuality was illegal in the past and many older men may still hide their true sexuality. Whilst lesbianism has never been illegal some lesbians may still remember when their relationships were seen as distasteful and were met with social disapproval (McMahon & Isaacs, 1997). Some older lesbians may have faced homophobic violence or religious condemnation and family rejection in the past because of their revealed sexuality (Deevey, 1990). To overcome these feelings some older lesbians may have hidden their true selves, some even marrying. As they age these hidden feelings may cause anger and resentment for a life not lived the way they may have desired. Nurses and care assistants are in an ideal position to help their patients explore their true sexuality in a safe, non judgemental atmosphere. McMahon & Isaacs (1997) recommend discussing the positive aspects taking place in today's society to benefit gay women, providing privacy and access to gay support groups. Waterhouse (1996) and Whittly (1997) argue that patients would prefer to have any discussion regarding sexuality and sexual concerns initiated by health care professionals, but research shows that nurses tend not to broach such subjects with their patients unless asked specifically.

Elderly women who may have committed themselves to a long term lesbian relationship can face legal problems due to their lack of status. In the United Kingdom lesbian relationships cannot be formally recognised through marriage, unlike heterosexual relationships. This can have legal consequences for the surviving partner in terms of life insurance and estate arrangements where the partners are not legally married (Heath, 1999). Elderly lesbians may have to deal with the additional emotional difficulties if family members contest their partner's will (Heath, 1999).

Many authors acknowledge that there are more older women than men and women may find it hard to find male partners (Brogan, 1996; Eliopoulos, 1993; Gibson, 1997a; Heath, 1999; Johnson, 1996; Russell, 1998). Gibson (1997a) argues that older women may find erotic love and fulfillment with female partners. Heath (1999) and Gibson (1997) acknowledge that many older people may choose to live alone, some may have lost loved ones earlier in their lives, and are content and happy.

Nurses and care assistants should remember that elderly lesbian or heterosexual sex is not just the physical act. It also encompasses an emotional well being of warmth, love, sharing, caring and closeness with another (Gibson, 1997a; Gibson 1997b; Johnson, 1996; Parke, 1991; Riley, 1999; Russell, 1998). Many elderly people will benefit from such meaningful and comforting relationships.

References

Brogan, M. (1996) The sexual needs of elderly people. Nursing Standard 10(24): 42–45.

Cole, J. (2001) Sexuality and older women. Nursing Older People 13(4): 6.

Deevey, S. (1990) Older lesbian women an invisible minority. Journal of Gerontological Nursing 16(5): 35–39.

Drench, M.E., Losee, R.H. (1996) Sexuality and sexual capacities in elderly people. Rehabilitation Nursing 21(3): 118–123.

Eliopoulos, C. (1993) Gerontological nursing. (3rd ed.). Philadelphia: J.B. Lippincott Company.

Ford, P. (1998) Sexuality and sexual health. Cited in H. Heath (2000). Sexuality in old age NT monographs No 40. London: NT books.

Gibson, H.B. (1997a) Love in later life. London: Peter Owen.

Gibson, H.B. (1997b) A little of what you fancy does you good: your health in later life. London: Third Age Press.

Grigg, E. (1999) Sexuality and older people. Elderly Care 11(7): 12–15.

Grigg, E. (2000) Sexually transmitted infections and older people. Elderly Care 12(1): 15–19.

Heath, H. (1999) Sexuality in old age. NT Monographs No 40. London: NT books.

Heath, H. (2000) Sexuality and continence in older women. Elderly Care 12(3): 32–34.

Heath, H., Schofield, I. (Eds) (1999) Healthy Ageing: Nursing Older People. London: Mosby.

Heath, H., White, I. (2001) Sexuality and older people: an introduction to nursing. Nursing Older People 13(4): 29–31.

Irwin, R. (2000) Treatments for patients with sexual problems. Professional Nurse 15(6): 360–364.

Johnson, B.K. (1996) Older adults and sexuality: A multidimensional perspective. Journal of Gerontological Nursing 22(2): 6–15.

Le Gallez, P. (Ed.) (1998) Rheumatology for Nurses: Patient Care. London: Whurr Publishers Ltd.

McMahon, C., Isaacs, R. (Eds) (1997) Care of the older person. Oxford: Blackwell Science.

Parke, F. (1991) Sexuality in later life. Nursing Times 87(50): 40–42.

Riley, A. (1999) Sex in old age: continuing pleasure or inevitable decline? Geriatric Medicine 29(3): 25–28.

Russell, P. (1998) Sexuality in the lives of older people. Nursing Standard 13(8): 49–53.

Thomas, L. (1999) Editorial. Elderly Care 11(7): 1.

Tortora, G.J., Grabowski, S.R. (1996) Principles of anatomy and physiology. (8th ed.). New York: Harper Collins College Publishers.

Tschudin, V. (Ed.) (2000) Counselling and older people. London: Age Concern England.

Waterhouse, J. (1996) Nursing practice related to sexuality: a review and recommendations. NT Research 1(6): 412–418.

Whittly, H. (1997) Your turn. Journal of Gerontological Nursing 23(10): 53–54.

Patient education

Penny Tremayne

> Max Barren is a 47-year-old married man who lives with his wife and three children aged 16, 12, and 8 years. He is a sales representative who travels countrywide. He enjoys spending time with his family and has recently returned from a holiday from the Far East. In his spare time he likes going to antique markets and car boot sales. Normally he only takes drugs (pain relief) if he has a headache, which is usually about twice a week. Ten days after returning from his holiday, Max is admitted to the local coronary care unit with a diagnosis of atrial fibrillation. This is treated successfully with cardioversion, however because of the risk of thrombi forming he is commenced on anti coagulant therapy, namely Warfarin tablets to be administered according to International Normalised Ratio (INR). Fully stabilised, Max is transferred to Sycamore ward from where he is due to be discharged home in 2 days. He is worried about taking the tablets and informs his named nurse that he would like to know a little bit more about them.

Question one: Briefly describe how learning needs are identified.

10 minutes

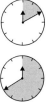

Question two: Discuss how a knowledge of learning theories can help you plan a teaching programme for Max.

40 minutes

Question three: How will you know if learning has occurred?

15 minutes

Time allowance: **65 minutes**

Answer to question one:
Briefly describe how learning needs are identified.

In this instance Max has perceived that he wants some knowledge, skills and understanding of how to correctly self administer warfarin tablets. This is known as a felt need.

Other needs can include:

- Normative need, this is where the need for learning is identified by the judgement of the healthcare professional.
- Expressed need, this is where the felt need has evolved and is expressed in words or action as a demand.
- Comparative needs, this is where there is an inequity in provision, one group when compared to another is found to be lacking or deficient in for example: services, resources education.

Naidoo and Wills (2000)

It is important that learning needs are identified within nursing assessment so that an individualised plan can be formulated, agreed upon and implemented.

Answer to question two:
Discuss how a knowledge of learning theories can help you plan a teaching programme for Max.

We all learn in different ways and it may initially be advised to discuss with Max and his family (if they want to be involved) how they best learn. Honey & Mumford (1998) identified four learning styles:

1. The activist – open minded, energetic, thrives on challenges of a new experience but can get bored with long term projects.
2. The pragmatist – practical, problem solving, enthusiastic to try out new ideas, experimental.
3. The theorist – thinks problems through in a logical step-by-step approach, perfectionist, systematic, analytical, objective.
4. The reflector – takes time to think, cautious, thoughtful.

After acknowledging individual learning styles, the approach to teaching should then be considered. There are two renowned teaching approaches: andragogy is considered as the art and science of helping adults to learn (Knowles, 1984) and pedagogy, the art and science of teaching children. Whichever teaching approach is preferred will directly influence the learning theory and strategies that will be used in teaching. Both approaches have differing underpinning assumptions of the learner (Fig. 9.1).

The learning theories that underpin the teaching process are: humanism behaviourism and cognitivism.

The humanistic learning theory (Rogers, 1983) is concerned with feelings and experiences which assist in the achievement of self actualisation. The qualities of this learning theory are: it involves the whole person, it is self initiated, it is pervasive and makes a difference in a person's attitude, it is evaluated by the learner (McKenna, 1995a).

Behavioural learning theory is based on the connection made between two events; a stimulus and a response (Howard, 1999):

- Classical conditioning, whereby a response can become conditioned by a stimulus
- Operant conditioning, whereby behaviour is directed by its consequences, in order to bring about desirable objectives, often a reward.

Cognitive learning theory is an internal purpose process that involves thinking, perception, organisation and insight (McKenna, 1995b). Perceptions are

Andragogy	Pedagogy
The learner is self directed	The learner is dependent
Values learner experience	Have less experience
Learners prefer to problem solve	Learners are motivated by external pressures
Student centred	Teacher led

Figure 9.1: Characteristics of andragogy and pedagogy.

organised into as simple a structure as possible so that meaning could be imposed, hence the phrase 'the whole is greater than the sum of its parts' was derived.

There is no right or wrong way to teach Max and his family; there may be elements of the teaching approaches and learning theories considered to be more appropriate and teaching may embrace the best qualities of all and therefore be eclectic. As a nurse it is important that the educational requirements of Max are detailed in an individualised care plan which comprises of an overall aim, or objective and specific steps, or learning outcomes to achieve the objective. Then the planning can consider:

- What needs to be taught
- When it needs to be taught
- How it is going to be taught, the teaching strategies that can be implemented
- Where it needs to be taught
- What resources will be required.

Answer to question three:
How will you know if learning has occurred?

A judgement has to be made on the effectiveness of Max's learning. There are a number of methods that could be considered:

- Elicit from Max himself if he feels learning has taken place
- Observation of Max self administering his medication, is he competent or not?
- Ask Max to complete a quiz.

In the short term, in a healthcare environment with support, it is relatively straightforward to assess learning, but it is more difficult in the long term. This may be judged by the monitoring of INR results. If there are any doubts that Max maybe unable to self administer his drugs and that his family feel unsure, then it should be considered that Max is referred to a District Nurse or to an anti coagulation specialist nurse to facilitate the educative process.

References

Honey, P., Mumford, A. Ch. 6. 'Setting the Scene for Learning Styles' in Downie, C., Basford, P. (1998) Teaching and Assessing in Clinical Practice: A Reader. (2nd ed.). London: Greenwich University Press.

Howard, S. Ch. 6. 'The process of learning' in Hinchliff, S. (1999) The Practitioner as Teacher. (2nd ed.). Edinburgh: Bailliere Tindall.

Knowles, M. (1984) Andragogy In Action: Applying Modern Principles of Adult Learning. San Francisco: Jossey Bass.

McKenna, G. (1995a) Learning theories made easy: humanism. Nursing Standard 9(31): 29–31.

McKenna, G. (1995b) Learning theories made easy: cognitivism. Nursing Standard 9(30): 25–28.

Naidoo, J., Wills, J. (2000) Health Promotion: Foundations for Practice. (2nd ed.). Edinburgh: Bailliere Tindall.

Rogers, C.R. (1983) Freedom to Learn for the 80s. Ohio: Merrill.

Further reading

Darbyshire, P. (1993) In defence of pedagogy: a critique of the notion of andragogy. Nurse Education Today 13: 328–335.

McKenna, G. (1995) Learning theories made easy: behaviourism. Nursing Standard 9(29): 29–31.

Milligan, F. (1995) In defence of andragogy. Nurse Education Today 15: 22–27.

Woodrow, P. (1993) A case for humanism in nurse education. Senior Nurse 13(5): 46–50.

Atrial fibrillation

Sam Parboteeah

Charity Chitembe is a 66-year-old widowed lady who lives in a bungalow on the outskirts of the city. She was born in Africa but has lived in this country for the last 30 years. She has three grown-up daughters, all married and living locally. They frequently visit their mother. Mrs Chitembe has had a history of hypertension and unstable angina and takes a beta-blocker but this has not stopped her from leading an active life.

Mrs Chitembe retired from her job as a secretary but has maintained contact with her work colleagues who visit her regularly for a chat. Mrs Chitembe has continued to remain active in the local African association and is involved in the annual local carnival.

Whilst she was attending the carnival she complained to her daughter that she was feeling breathless, giddy, was experiencing palpitations and chest pain. The emergency services were contacted and Mrs Chitembe was admitted to the coronary care unit. After an electrocardiograph a diagnosis of atrial fibrillation (AF) was made.

Question one: What is atrial fibrillation and list the possible causes of it.

20 minutes

Question two: Discuss the treatment of atrial fibrillation.

20 minutes

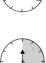

Question three: Describe the specific care that Mrs Chitembe will require for the first 24 hours.

20 minutes

Time allowance: **60 minutes**

Answer to question one:
What is atrial fibrillation and list the possible causes of it.

To understand the mechanism and characteristic of atrial fibrillation (AF), the normal mechanical and electrical activity will be described. In order for the heart to pump, it must first receive some form of electrical stimulation that will cause the cardiac muscles to contract. During a normal heart beat, an electrical impulse originates in the right atrium from the sino-atrial node (SA node) and travels simultaneously to the left atrium and down the atrioventricular node (AV node). The impulse slows briefly at the AV node and then continues to travel down a common pathway before dividing into the left and right bundle branches as shown in Figure 10.1.

Atrial fibrillation is an arrhythmia and is characterised by irregular and very rapid beating of the heart's atrial chambers and results when the electrical conduction system of the atria is disorganised and chaotic (Fig. 10.2), and the ventricular rate is usually about 120–150 per minute (Schamroth, 1990). The malfunction reduces cardiac output (Ott et al, 1997; Kilander et al, 1998) as a result of the loss of the atrial component of ventricular filling. These spasms may lead to reduced blood flow, blood clots, risk of stroke (Kannel et al, 1997) and even death.

The aetiology of atrial fibrillation is diverse and includes:

- advancing age, rheumatic and ischaemic heart disease, hypertension, diabetes, acute myocardial infarction, thyrotoxicosis, pulmonary embolism, alcohol, respiratory infections, cardiac surgery, chest injuries and idiopathic causes.

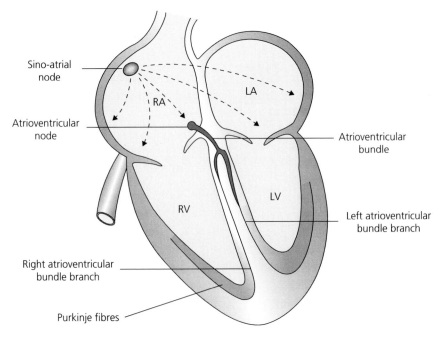

Figure 10.1: Conducting system of the heart.

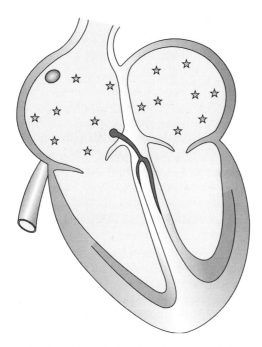

Figure 10.2: Atrial fibrillation – electrical system of atria is uncontrolled and disorganised.

Answer to question two:
Discuss the treatment of atrial fibrillation.

Current management of atrial fibrillation includes:

- Rate control – the goal of treatment is to keep the ventricular rate less than 90 beats per minute at rest. The doctor may prescribe intravenous digoxin which slows conduction across the AV node. Digoxin is less effective at controlling heart rate during exercise. Beta-blockers or calcium channel blockers may be prescribed as they are more effective at controlling heart rate at rest and on exercise (Segal et al, 2000).
- Rhythm control – sinus rhythm is often restored with medications by slowing the rate of conduction of electrical impulses, decreasing the excitability and automaticity of cardiac cells or by prolonging the refractory period of the cardiac muscle. Several medications may be used (Cordarone, disopyramide, procainamide).
- Cardioversion the restoration of the heart's normal sinus rhythm by delivery of a synchronized electric shock. If the AF is poorly tolerated or associated with adverse haemodynamic features (a heart rate greater than 200 beats per minute, systolic blood pressure less than 90 mmHg), urgent direct current (DC) cardioversion is indicated (Nolan et al, 1999). This intervention is thought to be useful because the restoration of sinus rhythm may reduce the risk of embolic complications, thereby obviating the need for long term coagulation, and the improvement in ventricular function.
- Antithrombotic treatment – patients who have an increased risk of embolic stroke should be treated with an anticoagulant. Based on the recommendation from SIGN (1999), Mrs Chitembe is in the high risk group of patients likely to be at significantly increased risk of stroke.

The next step in AF treatment may include:

- Ablation of specific arrhythmias
- Use of pacemakers

Whilst Mrs Chitembe is receiving treatment, she should be on continuous cardiac monitoring of heart rate, P-R interval, QRS duration and QT interval because many of the drugs used for pharmacologic cardioversion can cause further cardiac complications.

Answer to question three:
Describe the specific care that Mrs Chitembe will require for the first 24 hours.

Mrs Chitembe should be assessed for signs and symptoms of decreased cardiac output and heart failure. She will have her apical and radial pulse recorded. When the heart is in atrial fibrillation, not all cardiac contractions eject the same volume of blood. Hence, not all heart beats can be felt at the radial site. The rhythm may be irregular and therefore it is important to take the pulse for 1 minute. If any deficit is present between the apical and radial pulse, it should be recorded and reported to the medical staff.

Drugs should be administered as prescribed and Mrs Chitembe should be closely monitored because drugs may need to be titrated to achieve a therapeutic benefit. If any mechanical device is in use then check the correct administration rate. Mrs Chitembe will be attached to a cardiac monitor and she should be informed why she is attached to a monitor and not to be alarmed by it. Safety aspects should be explained. She should be assessed for any further giddiness, breathlessness and palpitations.

Mrs Chitembe's pain should be assessed and appropriate analgesics given. The effect of the drug should be monitored and if the patient is feeling nauseated, an anti-emetic may be given.

While Mrs Chitembe is on bed rest with limited mobility, she will require assistance with meeting her physical and psychological needs.

References

Kilander, L., Andren, B., Nyman, H., Lind, L., Boberg, M., Lithell, H. (1998) Atrial fibrillation is an independent determinant of low cognitive function. A cross sectional study in elderly men. Stroke 29: 1816–1820.

Kannel, W.B., Abbott, R.D., Savage, D., McNamara, P.M. (1997) Epidemiological features of chronic atrial fibrillation. N Engl Journal of Medicine 96: 310–316.

Nolan, J., Greenwood, J., Mackintosh, A. (1999) Cardiac Emergencies: a Pocket Guide. Oxford: Butterworth Heinemann.

Ott, A., Breteler, M.B., de Bruyne, M.C., van Harksamp, F., Grobbee, D.E., Hofman, A. (1997) Atrial fibrillation and dementia in a population based study. The Rotterdam study. Stroke 28: 316–321.

Schamroth, L. (1990) An Introduction to Electrocardiography. (7th ed.). Oxford: Blackwell Scientific Publications.

Segal, J.B., McNamara, R.L., Miller, M.R., et al (2000) The evidence regarding the drugs used for ventricular rate control. Journal of Family Practice 49: 47–49.

SIGN (1999) Atrial fibrillation: prophylaxis of systemic embolism. Scottish Intercollegiate Guidelines Network, pp. 18–22.

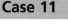

Endoscopy

Penny Harrison

Bevil Grenfell, is a 55-year-old married man with three teenage children. He works as a manager for a warehousing and packaging company. He is overweight at 90 kg, smokes five cigarettes daily (although he has reduced his consumption recently) and admits to taking no exercise at all. He states that he finds his job increasingly demanding with deadlines for big orders that are frequently problematic in terms of completion. To compensate for the stress Bevil experiences in his job, he socialises with his wife and friends at the local pub on Friday and Saturday evenings. Bevil usually consumes 6–8 pints of beer on these evenings and this is frequently followed by a large 'take-away' meal en route home. This is despite Bevil and his wife having had supper at home earlier in the evening. Bevil is also building a garage at home, which is behind schedule due to recent adverse weather conditions, where building work has not been possible. This is causing tension between Bevil and his wife, as the contents of the garage are being stored in the house, partially blocking the hall.

Bevil has recently been to see his General Practitioner (GP), complaining of a 6 month history of indigestion and acid reflux from his stomach. Prior to this, Bevil was managing his symptoms with 'over the counter' medicines to reduce the indigestion. These were only partially successful, so Bevil's GP has prescribed him a stronger antacid solution to ease his symptoms. Bevil has not had much relief from these medicines either, so has been referred to the local hospital's Endoscopy Unit for further investigations into his symptoms. Bevil requires an OGD (oesophagogastroduodenoscopy) to assess his symptoms.

Question one: What is an OGD and why would this test be required for Bevil?

10 minutes

Question two: What is the role of the nurse in preparing Bevil for OGD?

20 minutes

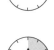

Question three: What do Bevil's symptoms suggest? Explain the factors or behaviours from Bevil's lifestyle that might be contributing to his symptoms.

20 minutes

Time allowance: **50 minutes**

Answer to question one:
What is an OGD and why would this test be required for Bevil?

D'Silva (1998) identifies oesophagogastroduodenoscopy (OGD) as a common test, accounting for about 70% of all investigations for the gastrointestinal tract. Endoscopy is based on the Greek word 'endo', which means to look in. Thus endoscopy enables the inside of the body to be looked at via a fibre-optic or video gastro scope, to view the upper gastrointestinal tract of the oesophagus, stomach and first part of the duodenum. The OGD allows for direct visualisation of the GI tract, plus examining the mucosa of the related organs and structures. Diagnostic procedures may include the taking of biopsies from the mucosa. For some patient therapeutic work such as dilatation of strictures may be performed. Reasons for performing an OGD include assessing for heartburn, acid regurgitation/reflux, strictures, erosions, ulceration, signs of haemorrhage or varices. Bevil has a history of acid reflux, which has not responded to medicines designed to reduce the acidity of stomach secretions, thus his symptoms warrant further investigation.

Answer to question two:
What is the role of the nurse in preparing Bevil for OGD?

The nurse has a multi-faceted role in preparing Bevil for OGD. These include:

- Information

Hughes (2002) discusses the role of information giving in anxiety reduction and reduction of potential complications for surgical patients. Whilst an OGD is not a surgical procedure, the principles translate well into the endoscopy setting. Hughes (2002) identifies how anxiety may manifest itself by accentuating the fear of an unknown environment by disturbing the patient's integrity outside the context of their usual activities of living. Thus Bevil requires details of what an OGD is, how it is to be performed and what happens after the test. Information should be tailored to the needs of the patient. For example using language like 'we are going to place a camera down your throat' may increase anxiety. Appropriate language such as 'we will be using a fibre optic endoscope that is the width of one of your fingers' gives patients correct information about the test to be undertaken. Crawford (1999) also suggests that information given pre procedure can be successfully reinforced to assist the patient with anxieties they may have.

- Consent

The Nursing and Midwifery Council (2002, para 3, page 4) Code of Professional Conduct states that the nurse must obtain consent before giving any treatment or care. In addition, Endoscopy Units will use formal consent forms for procedures of an invasive nature, based on the local Trust's consent policy. The nurse is well placed to ensure that Bevil has consented to the OGD, as well as ascertaining that he understands the nature of the investigation and has had opportunity to ask any questions relating to the OGD. This is required in written and verbal format and is recorded either on the consent form or the patient's notes that this information has been given. In addition, many policies require endoscopists to identify known risks and complications of procedures. For example, Bevil needs to know that the risk of perforation of the oesophagus for OGD is about one in one thousand patients (Cotton & Williams, 1996, 75). Based on this information, Bevil is able to give his informed consent to the procedure.

- Sedation

Local anaesthetic spray to the back of the throat is used for patients undergoing OGD. This is to allow for passage of the endoscope over the back of the throat into the oesophagus, preventing the gag reflex. Increasingly, sedation is not used for simple diagnostic OGD for many patients. This is because of the recognition of the risk of medicine induced respiratory depression. Where sedation is used, benzodiazepines are given in small doses titrated to patient response. The ideal being the patient who is 'consciously sedated', that is the patient is comfortable and sedated, but not anaesthetised and able to co-operate with the endoscopist and staff performing the procedure (Cotton & Williams, 1996, 25).

- Fasting

Bevil will be required to fast for 4–6 hours prior to the OGD or as per local policy. This is to allow the stomach to clear its contents so that the endoscopist has a clear view via the endoscope and can visualise the structures effectively as well as pass the endoscope safely through the upper part of the gastrointestinal tract.

Pre-OGD care/During-OGD care/Post-OGD care

The nurse is well placed to assist the endoscopist to perform the OGD for Bevil; this assistance is likely to encompass a number of aspects of care:

- Patient position and comfort – a well positioned, comfortable and relaxed patient will assist the endoscopist to pass the endoscope more easily, view the upper gastrointestinal (GI) tract clearly and complete the procedure in a safe and timely manner. Patients do not need to change into a hospital gown, but clothing should not be tight around the neck area.
- Recording of observations – baseline observations of temperature, pulse, blood pressure, respiration and oxygen saturation are recorded before OGD. Local units may vary in the level of monitoring. Observations will be repeated and these will be determined by the patient's response to the procedure.
- Labelling of any specimens taken – biopsies from the ODG require accurate labelling. This is to ensure that any future treatments required or diagnosis made from information gained from examination of the biopsies in the laboratories is given to the correct patient.
- Assisting to manage the patient's airway, clearing secretions via the mouthpiece – before the procedure commences a mouthpiece is inserted to allow the patient's airway to be maintained and for safe introduction of the endoscope. Dentures should be removed and any loose teeth noted. Throughout the procedure the nurse should ensure that the airway is free of secretions.
- Administration of oxygen via nasal cannulae – a low level of background oxygen is administered as prescribed. This is to assist with adequate oxygenation whilst the endoscope is in situ, occupying space in the oro-pharynx.
- Recovering the patient post procedure – if Bevil has had sedation he may be sleepy post procedure. He should continue to be nursed on his side until he is fully conscious to maintain his airway. Nurses should ensure patient safety and apply local protocols. He may be able to commence oral sips of water 20 minutes post procedure if he has had no sedation. This should be enough time for any locally applied anaesthetic to the pharynx to have worn off. Oral intake is gradually increased to free fluids and diet prior to discharge from the endoscopy unit.
- Follow up – Bevil will be told the results of his OGD after completion of the test. Depending upon the results, Bevil may be referred back to his GP for continuing care, or referred to a physician (gastroenterologist) or surgeon for further follow up or care. Bevil is likely to be prescribed medication for reduction of production of gastric acid in his stomach. The nurse needs to ensure that Bevil understands the nature of his medication and his requirements for continuing with the treatment regime, even if he feels his symptoms are resolving.

Answer to question three:
What do Bevil's symptoms suggest? Explain the factors or behaviours from Bevil's lifestyle that might be contributing to his symptoms.

Bevil's symptoms suggest that he is suffering from reflux of acidic stomach juices into the bottom end of the oesophagus, causing oesophagitis, as well as symptoms of indigestion and heart burn. The OGD will confirm this diagnosis and extent of damage that the reflux has caused. Bevil will require medication to assist with healing of inflamed mucosa in the gastrointestinal tract. However, the medication is only treating the symptom and not the cause of the reflux. The nurse is well placed to assess Bevil's lifestyle to assist with changes that may have a significant impact on reduction and management of his symptoms.

Part of the challenge for the nurse assessing Bevil, is that there appear to be multiple issues as listed below. This is also combined with habits that may be well established, as Bevil is middle aged. Thus the nurse will require support from Bevil's wife and family, consolidating this with written information in an appropriate format.

• Obesity/High fat diet

Obesity is a common problem in the developing countries, with the accumulation of body fat in excess of requirements for height and build. It is associated with the development of many health problems, symptoms and diseases (Gobbi & Torrance, 2000). For Bevil, his diet may directly contribute to his symptoms, as late night meals high in saturated fat intake may exacerbate acid reflux into the oesophagus. The nurse needs to weigh Bevil, complete a body mass index (BMI) calculation and nutritional assessment tool. The nurse can give general advice about the constituents of a healthy diet and may ask Bevil to keep a food diary. Referral to the dietician for specialist advice may be required. Bevil's wife should be actively involved with this process, especially if she predominantly cooks food for the family. Consideration of diet in the workplace, as well as part of leisure activities also needs attention.

• Smoking

Bevil has reduced his rate of cigarette smoking. He is to be commended for this, but should be encouraged to cease smoking altogether. Smoking is a major cause of ill health and is linked to a range of disorders and diseases (Edmond, 2000). For Bevil, smoking may cause changes in the mucosa of the upper gastrointestinal tract, predisposing him to development of ulceration. In combination with his history of acid reflux, this is to be taken seriously. The nurse can provide Bevil with a range of health promotion literature as well as information to local services and facilities such as smoking cessation clinics and prescriptions for nicotine replacement products.

• Alcohol

Alcohol is the commonest form of a psychoactive substance used by over 90% of adults in the United Kingdom. Bevil has a history a large amount of alcohol consumption at weekends. Alcohol is a direct irritant to the mucosa of the stomach and may be contributing to his symptoms of acid reflux. The nurse can advise Bevil and his wife about safe levels of alcohol intake, suggesting a range of alternative non-alcoholic and reduced alcoholic beverages and coping strategies to assist with alcohol reduction. Where services and facilities exist, referral to an alcohol advice or specialist nurse service may be required.

• Exercise

Taking part in forms of exercise, both from anecdotal reports as well as formal studies, demonstrate a positive impact on health. This may be associated with feelings of good health as well as the maintenance of cardiovascular fitness, stress reduction and weight control (Leefarr, 2000). For Bevil, exercise could be used for a range of facets of health promotion such as assisting with losing weight, stress reduction and better patterns of sleep. Family-centred exercise such as swimming, could also assist with relationships within the family unit and encourage fitness/improved health for the whole family. Greater participation in exercise may assist Bevil with his symptoms of acid reflux as his health status improves generally.

• Stress Management

Bevil encounters stress both at work and in the home environments. Stress is perceived differently by individuals, thus no standard plan of action is suitable for all patients. The nurse is well placed to informally assess Bevil's stress and give general advice about stress reduction and management techniques. From the nursing assessment, Bevil may require formal referral to specialists such as a psychologist or counsellor, either via his GP or occupational health department, who can advise further on stress reduction and management techniques.

References

Cotton, P., Williams, C. (1996) Practical Gastrointestinal Endoscopy. (4th ed.). Oxford: Blackwell Scientific.

Crawford, B. (1999) Highlighting the role of the peri-operative nurse: is pre-operative assessment necessary? British Journal of Theatre Nursing 3(4): 12–15.

D'Silva, J. (1998) Upper gastrointestinal endoscopy: gastroscopy. Nursing Standard 12(45): 49–56.

Edmond, C.B. (2000) Ch. 3. 'The Respiratory System' in Alexander, M., Fawcett, J., Runciman, P. (2000) Nursing Practice Hospital and Home: The Adult. Edinburgh: Churchill Livingstone.

Gobbi, M., Torrance, C. (2000) Ch. 21. 'Nutrition' in Alexander, M., Fawcett, J., Runciman, P. (2000) Nursing Practice Hospital and Home: The Adult. Edinburgh: Churchill Livingstone.

Hughes, S. (2002) The effects of giving patient pre-operative information. Nursing Standard 16(28): 33–37.

Leefarr, V. (2000) Ch. 17. 'Stress' in Alexander, M., Fawcett, J., Runciman, P. (2000) Nursing Practice Hospital and Home: The Adult. Edinburgh: Churchill Livingstone.

Nursing and Midwifery Council (2002) Code of Professional Conduct. London: NMC.

Further reading

Bruce, L., Finlay, T. (Eds) (1997) Nursing in Gastroenterology. Edinburgh: Churchill Livingstone.

Doughty, D. (1993) Gastroenterology Disorders. St. Louis: Mosby.

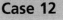

Deep vein thrombosis

Ricky Autar

Eleanor Tanner is a 67-year-old retired schoolteacher. She is currently taking Hormone Replacement Therapy (HRT) to slow down bone loss due to her established osteoporosis. She has limited mobility caused by her osteoporosis and bilateral varicose veins. Eleanor slowly mobilises about independently but uses a walking aid to steady her gait. Recently, Eleanor has been experiencing some difficulty in getting about her home and garden due to a swollen left foot. Homan's sign is positive. This type of pain elicited in the calf on dorsiflexion is thought to be a classical sign of deep vein thrombosis (DVT). The skin in the calf area is warm and tender to touch.

Following a domiciliary visit by her General Practitioner, Eleanor is suspected of having DVT and is referred to the anticoagulant outpatient clinic for investigation. An ultrasound confirms distal DVT of the calf and a regimen of anticoagulation commenced.

Question one: Explain the classic triad for the pathogenesis of DVT in Eleanor, as described by Virchow.

15 minutes

Question two: Why Eleanor is considered to be a risk subject for DVT?

10 minutes

Question three: What other known predisposing risk factors are associated with an increased risk for the development of DVT?

10 minutes

Question four: What are the clinical manifestations of DVT?

15 minutes

Question five: What are the investigations available to confirm Eleanor's suspected DVT?

10 minutes

Question six: What complications Eleanor is likely to develop as a result of her DVT?

10 minutes

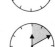

Question seven: Explain how Eleanor could have been protected against DVT.

10 minutes

Question eight: What treatment would be initiated for Eleanor's DVT?

10 minutes

Time allowance: **90 minutes**

Answer to question one:
Explain the classic triad for the pathogenesis of DVT in Eleanor, as described by Virchow.

Our understanding of the pathogenesis of DVT is derived from the pioneering work of Rudolf Virchow (1821–1902). The triad of factors that are associated with DVT are:

1. Changes in the vessel wall due to damage to the endothelium lining the vessel. Trauma, fracture, thermal injury, phlebitis, varicose veins, surgical procedures and instrumentation may cause injury to the endothelium. Venous stasis and venodilation can also cause microtears to the endothelium.
2. Changes to the blood flow due to venous stasis. Immobility is one of the major contributors of venous stasis. Venous stasis causes abnormal blood flow in the valve pockets, which are potential sites for thrombi formation.
3. Changes in the composition of blood due to hypercoagulability. Increased platelet activity and/or a decrease in physiological anticoagulant and fibrinolytic activity cause increased coagulation. Fibrinolysis is a system that is concerned with the dissolution of blood clot by the active enzyme plasmin.

Answer to question two:
Why Eleanor is considered to be a risk subject for DVT?

Risk factors are those characteristics or events that have been shown to increase the probability of becoming diseased. Eleanor has the following characteristics, which are recognised risk factors for DVT:

Advancing age: There is a linear relationship between the incidence of DVT and increasing age. DVT is uncommon in children and risk increases after the age of 40 (THRiFT, 1998). 50 per cent of DVT occurs in the 60–80 age group (Samama et al, 1993). Physiologically, advanced age is associated with decreased muscle calf pump, predisposing to venous stasis. Dilation of the deep vein due to stasis may cause microtears in the endothelium (Caprini et al, 1991).

Immobility: Eleanor has limited mobility due to her osteoporosis and varicose veins. There is a striking association between immobility and the incidence of DVT (Warlow, 1978; Kierkegaard et al, 1987). Immobility causes impairment of the venous pump and stasis which is one of the three elements of Virchow's triad predisposing to DVT.

Varicose veins: Anatomically, veins have semilunar valves, occurring at regular intervals. The valves are arranged so that blood flow is towards the heart. Stretching the veins increases their cross-sectional areas, but the valves do not increase in size. As a result, the valves do not close completely. When this develops, the pressure in the veins of the leg increases still more owing to the failure of the venous pump. Consequently, venous stasis is inevitable. Varicosities of the veins cause phlebitis, leading to increased risk of DVT.

HRT: There is little doubt that HRT has numerous long-term benefits in menopausal women. These include the prevention of osteoporosis and reduction in cardiovascular diseases such as myocardial infarction (Morris, 1998). However, HRT has been linked with the occurrence of DVT (THRiFT, 1998). Daly et al (1996) and Jick et al (1996) have both demonstrated that the current use of HRT is associated with an increased relative risk of 3.5 and 3.6, respectively, of developing DVT. From a biological perspective, HRT predisposes to hypercoagulability in the genesis of DVT.

Answer to question three:
What other known predisposing risk factors are associated with an increased risk for the development of DVT?

Other risk factors that predispose to DVT are listed below:

- Obesity
- Oral contraceptives
- Pregnancy and puerperium
- Thrombophilia
- Trauma
- Surgery
- Current high risk diseases such as ulcerative colitis, polycythaemia, myocardial infarction, chronic heart diseases, varicose veins, malignancy, CVA and previous DVT.

Data: Autar, 1996, 1998, 2002

Answer to question four:
What are the clinical manifestations of DVT?

The clinical signs and symptoms of DVT are notoriously unreliable and may mimic other clinical conditions. DVT is often asymptomatic and clinical signs and symptoms are present in only one third of patients (Caprini & Natonson, 1989). The so-called classic manifestation associated with the diagnosis of DVT is outlined below:

- Asymmetrical ankle oedema.
- Increased diameter of one calf, ankle or thigh in relation to the other.
- Loss of concavity of the malleolar space in one leg.
- Heavy and dull aching pain.
- Low grade fever.
- Homans' sign positive in one third of patients. This is the elicitation of pain in the calf on dorsiflexion.
- Dilation of the superficial veins.
- Phlegmasia alba dolens (painful white inflammation) or 'milk leg'. This is also called iliofemoral thrombophlebitis. It is caused by major venous thrombosis involving the deep veins of the thigh and pelvis. Skin blanching occurs when the interstitial pressure exceeds the capillary pressure.
- Phlegmasia cerulea dolens (painful blue inflammation). This is caused by total occlusion of deep venous circulation leading to the danger of limb loss due to cessation of arterial flow. Venous gangrene is likely to occur if adequate treatment is not initiated to restore the blood flow.
- Affected extremity is warmer to touch than the other unaffected extremity.

Answer to question five:
What are the investigations available to confirm Eleanor's suspected DVT?

As her clinical sign and symptom of painful swollen left leg is non-specific and clinical assessment is full of pitfalls (Redman, 1988), Eleanor has had to undergo some objective investigations to confirm the suspected DVT. The following investigations are available to diagnose DVT:

* Venography
* Impedance Phlethysmography (IPG)
* Compression Ultrasonography (US)
* Magnetic Resonance Imaging (MRI)
* D-Dimer measurement.

Venography: This is an invasive procedure whereby a contrast medium is injected into the dorsal pedal vein, allowing for the direct visualisation of the venous system to detect occlusive and non-occlusive thrombi. Any thrombus isolated will show up as intraluminal filling. Contrast venography is the gold standard for evaluating patients with suspected DVT primarily due to its long history and general accuracy in terms of positive and negative findings (Redman, 1988). Because this invasive procedure is associated with technical difficulties and potential allergic reactions due to the irritation of the endothelium, it has been essentially replaced by sensitive and safe non-invasive techniques.

Impedance Phlethysmography (IPG): This involves inflation of proximal thigh cuff, which obstructs venous outflow to allow maximal distal filling. The cuff is then deflated and alteration in flow is measured. Normal test indicates rapid outflow. The presence of occlusion reveals a prolongation of the outflow wave. IPG is non-invasive, risk free, relatively inexpensive but is less accurate for detecting calf DVT.

Compression Ultrasonography (CUS): This is a non-invasive technique that uses high resolution colour doppler to create two-dimensional images of the blood vessels. Pressure is applied to detect change in venous compressibility and flow produced by intra-luminal thrombi based on high frequency sound waves. Failure of total compressibility of the vein indicates the presence of a thrombus.

Magnetic Resonance Imaging (MRI): It is the diagnostic test of choice for suspected iliac vein or inferior vena caval thrombosis (Schreiber, 2000). MRI uses a large magnet, radio waves and a computer to scan the body and produce detailed pictures. A radionuclide is tagged to a small molecule that localises to a part of a thrombus.

D-Dimer: One shortcoming of available non-invasive tests to confirm suspected DVT is the occurrence of false positive outcome (Wells et al, 1995). False positive refers to patients with a positive diagnosis for the disease but who do not have it. To reduce the number of false positives and support the non-invasive techniques, D-Dimer is measured. D-Dimer is a specific degradation product of crosslinked fibrin. It is released when the fibrinolytic system for the dissolution of clot attacks the fibrin matrix of fresh venous thrombi. D-Dimer is not the ultimate test but when combined with non-invasive techniques for suspected DVT, it guides decision making as to whether to or not to treat the patient.

Answer to question six:
What complications Eleanor is likely to develop as a result of her DVT?

In the immediate unresolved course, DVT is a precursor of Pulmonary Embolism (PE) a potentially lethal and acute complication. The rate of fatal PE is estimated at 60 per 100,000 of the general population (International Consensus Statement, 1997). In the long-term sequelae, Eleanor faces an uncertain future as the DVT can complicate into Post Phlebitis Syndrome (PPS) (Dalen et al, 1986). PPS is a chronic disabling condition, characterised by phlebitis, leg pigmentation and ulceration. Long term complication of PPS commonly results in chronic venous leg ulceration (Nelzen et al, 1991). Eleanor also may have recurrence of the DVT. Patients with previous DVT are 8 times more likely to develop recurrence of the condition compared to patients without a previous history (Samama et al, 1993).

Answer to question seven:
Explain how Eleanor could have been protected against DVT.

DVT is very preventable (Anderson & Wheeler, 1995). Primary prevention is concerned with the identification of patients like Eleanor who are at risk, followed by the administration of the most appropriate venous thrombo-prophylaxis. This can be achieved by proactively assessing patients, using a DVT risk calculator. The Thrombosis Risk Factor (TRF) (Caprini et al, 1991) and the Autar DVT scale (Autar, 1996) are two risk assessment tools available to identify patients into risk categories.

The most recently revalidated Autar DVT scale (2002) is illustrated in Figure 12.1. Stratification of patients into risk categories facilitates the choice of the most appropriate prophylaxis as tabled below:

Risk category	Recommended DVT prophylaxis
Low risk	Encourage mobilisation + Active and passive exercises + Graduated compression stockings
Moderate risk	Early mobilisation + Graduated compression stockings + Low dose heparin or Low molecular weight heparin or Intermittent pneumatic compression
High risk	Graduated compression stockings + Adjusted dose of heparin or Low molecular weight heparin + Intermittent pneumatic compression, except for open limb injury.

Venous thromboprophylaxis strategies

THRiFT, 1998

Client profiles in nursing: adult & the elderly 2

Name of patient: Date of Birth: Age: Diagnosis: Type of Admission:

Age Group	Score
10-30	0
31-40	1
41-50	2
51-60	3
61-70	4
71+	5

Mobility	Score
Ambulant	0
Limited: Uses aids self	1
Very Limited: Needs help	2
Chairbound	3
Complete Bedrest	4

Build / Body Mass Index (BMI) BMI= wt (kg) / ht (m)2	Score
Underweight BMI: 16-19	0
Average BMI: 20-25	1
Overweight BMI: 26-30	2
Obese BMI: 31-40	3
Very Obese BMI: 41+	4

Special Risk Category	Score
Oral Contraceptive 20-35 yrs	1
Oral Contraceptive 35+ yrs	2
Hormone Replacement Therapy	2
Pregnancy & Puerperium	3
Thrombophilia	4

Trauma (Score item(s) only preoperatively)	Score
Head Injury	1
Chest Injury	1
Spinal Injury	2
Pelvic Injury	3
Lower Limb Injury	4

Surgery (Score only one appropriate item)	Score
Minor Surgery <30 mins	1
Planned Major Surgery	2
Emergency Major Surgery	3
Thoracic Surgery	3
Gynaecological Surgery	3
Abdominal Surgery	3
Urological Surgery	3
Neurosurgery	3
Orthopaedic Surgery (Below Waist)	4

Current High Risk Diseases: (Score all appropriate item(s))	Score
Ulcerative Colitis	1
Polycythaemia	2
Varicose Veins	3
Chronic Heart Disease	3
Acute Myocardial Infarction	4
Malignancy (Active Cancer)	5
CVA	6
Previous DVT	7

Any other assessment instructions:

Contra-indication to anticoagulants: Yes ☐   No ☐
If Yes, please specify:

ASSESSMENT: within 24 hours of admission.

SCORING: Ring out appropriate item(s) from each category column, add scores and record below:

Total Score [   ]   Assessor: Date:

ASSESSMENT PROTOCOL

Score Range	Risk Categories
≤10	Low risk
11-14	Moderate risk
≥15	High risk

VENOUS THROMBOPROPHYLAXIS

Low risk: Early ambulation + Graduated Compression Stockings.
Moderate risk: Graduated Compression Stockings + Low-Dose Heparin or Intermittent Sequential Compression.
High risk: Graduated Compression Stockings + Low-Dose Heparin + Intermittent Sequential Compression.

Recommended by:
International Consensus Statement 1997 & 2001
THRiFT Consensus Group 1998.

© R. Autar 2002.

Figure 12.1: Autar Risk Assessment Scale revalidated.

Answer to question eight:
What treatment would be initiated for Eleanor's DVT?

Anticoagulation remains the mainstay of initial treatment of DVT. The primary aim of treating DVT is to prevent PE, reduce morbidity and prevent/minimise the long term complication of post phlebitis syndrome.

Traditional management of an acute episode of DVT necessitates admission to hospital and anticoagulation with Unfractionated Heparin (UFH). In an average adult, an initial bolus of 5000–10,000 units is administered intravenously. This is followed by continuous intravenous infusion at 1000 units hourly. Partial Activated Thromboplastin time (APTT) is estimated and maintained at 1.5–2 times control. Warfarin overlaps with heparin for 4–5 days because of delayed onset of action of warfarin. Initially 10–15 mg of Warfarin is given orally followed by a maintenance dose of 2.5–7.5 mg daily, depending on an internationally normalised ratio (INR) of 2–3.

However, with the advent of Low Molecular Weight Heparin (LMWH) patients with confined proximal DVT are safely and effectively treated as outpatients or at home (Levine et al, 1996; Deagle, 1998). LMWH obviates the need for intravenous infusion and serial monitoring of APPT as required for UFH. Patients who are treated with LMWH are instructed to initiate therapy with 5 mg Warfarin the next day. LMWH and Warfarin are overlapped for about 5 days until INR is within the therapeutic range of 2–3.

References

Anderson, F.A., Wheeler, H.B. (1995) Venous thromboembolism: risk factors and prophylaxis. Clinics in Chest Medicine 16(2): 235–251.

Autar, R. (1996) Nursing assessment of clients at risk of deep vein thrombosis (DVT): the Autar DVT scale. Journal of Advanced Nursing 23: 763–770.

Autar, R. (1998) Deep Vein Thrombosis: the Silent Killer. Wiltshire: Quay Book, Mark Allen Publishing.

Autar, R. (2002) Advancing clinical practice in the management of deep vein thrombosis (DVT). Development, application and evaluation of the DVT scale. PhD thesis, De Montfort University, Leicester, England.

Caprini, J.A., Natonson, R.A. (1989) Postoperative deep vein thrombosis: current clinical considerations. Seminars in Thrombosis and Haemostasis 15(3): 244–249.

Caprini, J.A., Arcelus, J.I., Hasty, J.H. et al (1991) Clinical assessment of venous thromboembolic risk in surgical patients. Seminars in Thrombosis and Haemostasis 17(3): 304–312.

Dalen, J.E., Paraskos, J.A., Ockene, I.S. et al (1986) Venous thromboembolism. Scope of the problem. Chest (Suppl) 371S–373S.

Daly, E., Vessey, M.P., Painter, R. et al (1996) Risk of venous thromboembolism in users of hormone replacement therapy. Lancet 348: 977–980.

Deagle, J. (1998) Hospital at home. Deep vein thrombosis: low molecular weight heparin anticoagulant therapy. Primary Health Care 8(9): 23–25.

International Consensus Statement (1997) Prevention of Venous Thromboembolism. Med-Orion Publishing Company.

International Consensus Statement (2001) Prevention of Venous Thromboembolism. International Angiology 20(1): 1–37.

Jick, H., Derby, I.E., Myers, M.W. (1996) Risk of hospital admission for idiopathic venous thromboembolism among users of postmenopausal oestrogens. Lancet 248: 981–983.

Kierkegaard, A., Lars, N., Olson, C.G. et al (1987) Incidence of DVT in bedridden non-surgical patients. Acta Med Scand 222: 409–414.

Levine, M., Gent, M., Hirsch, J. et al (1996) A comparison of low molecular weight heparin administered primarily at home with unfractionated heparin administered in the hospital for proximal deep vein thrombosis. The New England Journal of Medicine 336(11): 677–681.

Morris, E. (1998) HRT: still a role in CVD. Geriatric Medicine 28(8): 27–31.

Nelzen, O., Bergqvist, D., Lindhagen, A. (1991) Leg ulcer aetiology. A cross sectional population study. Journal of Vascular Surgery 14: 557–564.

Redman, H.C. (1988) Deep vein thrombosis: is contrast venography still the diagnostic 'gold standard'. Radiology 168: 277–278.

Samama, M.M., Simmoneau, G., Wainstein, J.P. (1993) Sirius study. Epidemiology of risk factors of deep venous thrombosis (DVT) of the lower limb in community practice. Thrombosis Haemostasis 68: 763.

Schreiber, D. (2000) Deep venous thrombosis and thrombophlebitis. Emedicne.com/emerg/topic 122.htm.

THRiFT (1998) Risk of and prophylaxis for venous thromboembolism in hospital patients. Phlebology 13: 87–97.

Virchow, R. (1846) Uber die verfpfung der lungenarterie. Nue Notisen und Geb D Natur Heilk. 36: 26.

Warlow, C (1978) Venous thromboembolism after stroke. Am Heart Journal 96(3): 283–285.

Wells, P.S., Brill-Edwards, P., Stevens, P. et al (1995) A novel and rapid whole blood assay for D-Dimer in patients with clinically suspected deep vein thrombosis. Circulation 91: 2184–2187.

Suicide

Chris Buswell

Mr Wilfred Underwood is a 72-year-old retired dairy farmer. He lives in his old farm house with his wife, Gladys, who is 68 years old. His son now runs the farm, and lives in a nearby bungalow, on his land, that his father had built as a wedding gift. Mrs Gladys Underwood has terminal breast cancer. She is being cared for by Mr Underwood, their daughter-in-law Heather, and the district nursing team. Their regular district nurse, Sheila, has referred Mrs Underwood to the Macmillan nursing team in preparation for the time when Mrs Underwood will require more specialist palliative care. At present Mrs Underwood's pain is controlled by morphine sulphate tablets. However Mr Underwood feels that Mrs Underwood is in more pain than she discloses and discusses this with the district nurse in the kitchen whilst his wife is resting in the lounge.

'She's getting weaker by the day, Sheila. I'm sure she's putting on a brave face just for me. Those tablets are just not working, I hate to see her in pain and suffering so,' sighed Mr Underwood.

'When I chatted to Gladys she said she doesn't have any pain,' replied Sheila. 'She did say she feels so sleepy most of the time though. What makes you say she's in pain?'

'Oh I know my wife well enough by now,' smiled Mr Underwood grimly. 'She's the one who's kept this family and farm going, especially when we had the threat of cattle infection. Always had a brave fearless face, but underneath she's just as pained and worried as the rest of us. I've seen enough dying cows in my day to recognise the signs of pain. I've helped end some of them of their pain. Gladys is in pain all right, and there's not much I can do about it. She wants to die here on the farm, because that's been our life together. I can't help Robert run the farm as well as I could because of my hips. When I lose Gladys there won't be much left for me. I want to die here too. I love this farm and I love Gladys. I don't want to be apart from her. Nor will I see her suffering so, if you and the doctors can't stop her suffering I know I can. And we'll be going together.' Mr Underwood stared bleakly at Sheila ...

Question one: Discuss suicide in the elderly, relating answers to Mr and Mrs Underwood.

Time allowance: **1 hour**

Answer to question one:
Discuss suicide in the elderly, relating answers to
Mr and Mrs Underwood.

Many authors describe differing rates of suicide in the elderly (those over the age of 65 years). Eliopoulos (1993) describes the rate as 23% of all suicides being in this age group. Duffy (1997) states that this is slightly higher at a quarter of all suicides, whilst Wade (1994) defines the rate as over 50% higher than the average population.

Common forms of suicide adopted by the elderly include self starvation (Eliopoulos, 1993; Heath & Schofield, 1999) and medication over-dosage (Bates & Dines, 1999; Eliopoulos, 1993; Duffy, 1997). Commonly the elderly will use medications such as sedatives, anti-depressants and analgesics since these are readily prescribed for chronic health conditions (Bates & Dines, 1999).

Whilst people may be appalled when younger people commit suicide, there can be resigned acceptance when an older person commits suicide (Duffy, 1997). This may go some way to explain why older people are at a greater risk of repeating parasuicide (attempted suicide) or completing suicide (Bates & Dines, 1999).

Talk of suicide may be a sign of desperation and a cry for help; a way out of a situation with which the individual cannot cope (Eliopoulos, 1993; Roberts, 1996; Tschudin, 1999). Two thirds of successful suicides had tried or had told someone of their intentions (Duffy, 1997). Sheila, the district nurse should discuss openly and empathically with Mr Underwood his feelings of suicide and whether he feels that he could be depressed. A risk assessment should be performed and a referral, to a mental health service such as the community psychiatric nurse, should follow (Duffy, 1997; Roberts, 1996). Sheila should encourage Mr Underwood to visit his general practitioner (Roberts, 1996). Sheila should discuss Mr Underwood's thoughts with her nursing team. To show their support and to monitor the behaviour of Mr Underwood the nursing team should increase their visits to Mr and Mrs Underwood. Mead, Bower and Gask (1997) argue that district nurses have the opportunity to increase their assessment and support of people suffering psychological disorders of old age.

Studies have demonstrated a relationship between depression and suicide, especially late diagnosed depression (Duffy, 1997; Eliopoulos, 1993; Heath & Schofield, 1999; Roberts, 1996). It could be argued that, rather than feeling depressed, someone like Mr Underwood, may have feelings of hopelessness. Should such feelings of hopelessness continue then individuals may feel that suicide is the answer to end their despair (Cutcliffe, 1998; Duffy, 1997; Roberts, 1996).

Not all older people who commit suicide will have openly talked about their fears or their intended actions. Some may have suicidal thoughts or commit suicide on significant dates, such as an anniversary of a bereavement (Duffy, 1997). Others may exhibit the classical behaviour of someone intending to commit suicide which is outlined in Figure 13.1 (Duffy, 1997).

Older men, like Mr Underwood, are more at risk of attempted suicide (parasuicide) and suicide (Eliopoulos, 1993; Fillit & Picariello, 1998; Heath &

Schofield, 1999; Roberts, 1996; Wade, 1994). Being a farmer, Mr Underwood is at greater risk of suicide than many since farmers have been ranked as fourth per proportional rate at risk of committing suicide (Hughes, 1996), this is often seen as being due to them having easy access to potential and lethal means (Hughes, 1996; Roberts, 1996). Approximately 70 farmers a year take their own lives (Hampshire, 2001).

Bates and Dines (1999), De La Cour (2000), Duffy (1997), Heath and Schofield (1999) and Roberts (1996) urge nurses to be aware of patients who are in the risk categories outlined in Figure 13.2.

- Giving away possessions
- Changing a will
- Preoccupation with religion

Figure 13.1: Mr and Mrs Underwood.

- People who have recently moved home or relocated and possibly lost close social contacts
- The recently bereaved, especially those who have lost a partner
- Someone who has experienced the breakup of his or her family
- The isolated
- Someone having to cope with a protracted, or debilitating illness or physical health problem, or in the case of Mr Underwood, the effects of his wife's illness
- Chronic or unrelieved pain such as Mrs Underwood is experiencing
- Someone with low self esteem, role/job loss (e.g. Mr Underwood who is unable to help on the farm), or depression
- A carer, such as Mr Underwood
- Someone with mental health problems
- Someone who has the knowledge and means to fatally self harm

Figure 13.2: Mr and Mrs Underwood.

References

Bates, N., Dines, A. (1999) The risks of poisoning in later life. Elderly Care 11(3): 8–11.
Cutcliffe, J.R. (1998) Hope, counselling and complicated bereavement reactions. Journal of Advanced Nursing 28(4): 754–761.
De La Cour, J. (2000) Suicide in the ward setting. Nursing Times 96(40): 39–40.
Duffy, D. (1997) Suicide in later life: how to spot the risk factors. Nursing Times 93(11): 56–57.
Eliopoulos, C. (1993) Gerontological Nursing. (3rd ed.). Philadelphia: J.B. Lippincott Company.

Fillit, H.M., Picariello, G. (1998) Practical Geriatric Assessment. London: Greenwich Medical Media Ltd.

Hampshire, M. (2001) We're crying with them. Nursing Times 97(14): 14.

Heath, H., Schofield, I. (Eds) (1999) Healthy Ageing: Nursing Older People. London: Mosby.

Hughes, H. (1996) Preventing suicide among isolated farmers. Community Nurse 2(6): 12–13.

Mead, N., Bower, P., Gask, L. (1997) Emotional problems in primary care: what is the potential for increasing the role of nurses? Journal of Advanced Nursing 26(5): 879–890.

Roberts, D. (1996) Suicide prevention by general nurses. Nursing Standard 10(17): 30–33.

Tschudin, V. (Ed.) (1999) Counselling and Older People. London: Age Concern.

Wade, B. (1994) Depression in older people: a study. Nursing Standard 8(40): 29–35.

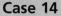

Overdose

Penny Tremayne

Joshua Hewitt is a 22-year-old final year media studies student who shares a rented terrace house with three other students. Since starting university Joshua has worked in a pub for four evenings a week but recently due to increasing debt he has taken on another part time job as an office cleaner.

This has left Joshua with little time for his studies. He has failed his last two pieces of assessed work and is behind time with the writing of his research dissertation. He was not short listed for a job he had applied for. On graduation he wants to return to his home town some 300 miles away to spend more time with his family and girlfriend. Joshua's father has become ill and the long distance relationship with his girlfriend has become strained.

Recently Joshua has lost weight. He has become more introverted and is prone to swings in mood. He feels anxious, panics and thinks that the world is collapsing in on him. One morning, one of the house mates, Steve finds Joshua smelling of alcohol, barely rousable on the sofa. Steve becomes further concerned when on the kitchen table he finds a half empty bottle of cough linctus and two empty ten tablet blister packs of paracetamol.

Alarmed that Joshua may have taken an overdose he phones for an emergency ambulance.

Question one: Explore the medical and nursing management that Joshua will require.

40 minutes

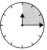

Question two: Provide an overview of what advice and support Joshua will require following his recovery.

15 minutes

Time allowance: **55 minutes**

Client profiles in nursing: adult & the elderly 2

Answer to question one:
Explore the medical and nursing management that Joshua will require.

Interventions will depend on the stage of overdose and clinical manifestations which indicate the extent of damage to the liver (Budden & Vink, 1996). An attempt at detailing the substance(s) taken should be obtained, as should the time of the overdose and the number of tablets and the quantity of alcohol consumed. Presenting within 15–24 hours of ingestion, Joshua's medical management as recommended by National Poisons Information Service (1999) guidelines includes:

- The immediate commencement of N-acetylcysteine (NAC) for example (Parvolex): 150 mg/kg intravenous (IV) infusion in 200 millilitres (ml) 5% dextrose over 15 minutes then,
- 50 mg/kg IV infusion in 500 ml 5% dextrose over 4 hours then,
- 100 mg/kg IV infusion in 1000 ml 5% dextrose over 16 hours.
- Urgent blood tests should be taken to estimate plasma paracetamol concentration and to determine the International Normalised Ratio (INR), plasma creatinine and alanine aminotransferase (ALT). Other blood tests may also be taken as there is a risk that Joshua may be more severely poisoned and consequently at greater risk of developing serious liver damage as he has presented some estimated 15 hours or longer after ingestion. These may include: plasma bicarbonate, and venous blood acid-base balance.
- Depending on the results of the plasma paracetamol concentration treatment NAC can be discontinued if identified as within normal limits and if there is no abnormality of the INR, plasma creatinine or ALT. It must continue if the results are abnormal or if Joshua is symptomatic. It would be usual to contact the National Poisons Information Service (NPIS).
- If the patient is asymptomatic and the repeat blood results are normal they can be discharged from medical care with the warning to return to hospital immediately if he develops vomiting or abdominal pain (NPIS guidelines, 1999). In Joshua's case he would remain in hospital as he is not responding to verbal commands.

So far most of the medical management has focused overtly on the physical aspects; another significant factor in the management of a patient like Joshua is psychological assessment. When Joshua is awake he will be seen by the psychiatrist on call for assessment and his/her recommendations will also influence the planning of Joshua's discharge.

Nursing management will focus on the monitoring of vital signs such as temperature, pulse, respiratory rate and blood pressure as well as neurological observations, maintenance of airway, administration of drug regime, monitoring of fluid balance, assessment of nutritional status, assessment of skin integrity, monitoring of daily weight and observation for potential alteration in tissue perfusion, monitoring for signs of potential bleeding (haemorrhage) (Budden & Vink, 1996). As a nurse you should be aware of the symptoms for early and late clinical manifestations of liver damage:

- Gastrointestinal cramping
- Nausea and vomiting
- Jaundice
- Hypoglycaemia
- Abdominal pain
- Ascites
- Diarrhoea
- Reduced urine output
- Bleeding.

The psychological ramifications should be considered. Nurses should be non judgemental and only gently try and elicit information from Joshua on an ongoing basis. Joshua's non-verbal cues should be continually assessed. Joshua should be nursed where he can be continually observed.

As a nurse it is important to recognise that although Joshua's condition may appear improved, liver damage is a slow process and deterioration would happen over a number of days.

Answer to question two:
Provide an overview of what advice and support Joshua will require following his recovery.

Joshua will only be discharged if he is medically and psychologically fit. If there is any concern that Joshua is not able to cope he may be transferred to a mental health unit. The advice and support that would be offered is as follows:

- To avoid hepatotoxic chemicals such as paracetamol and alcohol until the liver is completely recovered.
- Refer and attend a counselling service.
- Attend out-patient clinics so that blood clotting can be monitored.
- In the event of any of these presenting then contact a Doctor as soon as possible: weight gain; ascites, peripheral oedema; excessive bruising; jaundice and/or dark urine; influenzae like symptoms such as fever.
- Academic support from the University.
- Social support including family.

References

Budden, L., Vink, R. (1996) Paracetamol overdose: pathophysiology and nursing management. British Journal of Nursing 5(3): 145–152.
National Poisons Information Service (1999) Guidelines for the management of acute paracetamol overdosage. Paracetamol Information Centre.

Further reading

Roberts, D., MacKay, G. (1999) A nursing model of overdose assessment. Nursing Times 95(3): 58–60.
Seddon, C. (1994) Paracetamol overdose. Surgical Nurse 7(6): 15–19.
Tempowki, J. (2000) Gut decontamination and poisoning. Emergency Nurse 8(6): 22–28.

Useful address

Paracetamol Information Centre
78 Farquhar Road
London
SE19 1LT
Website: http://www.pharmweb.net/paracetamol.html

Acute bowel obstruction

Sam Parboteeah

Mrs White is a 54-year-old married lady who lives with her husband in a cottage. They have three grown up sons; one son lives locally and the other two sons live overseas. Mrs White has had abdominal surgery 2 years ago. Mrs White worked as a primary school teacher but has given up work following her surgery as she became exhausted at the end of a day. She has been managing to maintain an active life at home and also spending more time doing her gardening which she enjoys. Over a 24 hour period, Mrs White has been experiencing pain of a colicky nature in the abdominal region. She did not want to contact the General Practitioner (GP) as she hoped the pain would resolve after taking non prescription indigestion remedies. After her evening meal, she was resting. Unfortunately, her pain became unbearable, and she contacted her GP for an emergency domiciliary visit. Whist she was waiting for the GP to arrive, she vomited her meal, was sweating profusely and became very pale. She was tearful and frightened as she was alone at the time. On examination, the GP suspected an acute bowel obstruction and arranged for her to be admitted to the hospital as an emergency.

On admission to hospital she was examined by the surgeon and the diagnosis was confirmed. The patient was informed that she would require surgery. As Mrs White was dehydrated an intravenous infusion was set up and commenced immediately. An opiate was administered to control the pain and a nasogastric tube was inserted to empty the stomach. Mrs White went to theatre as an emergency and had a resection of the jejunum.

Question one: Discuss the physiological changes that occur in the intestine as a result of obstruction.

25 minutes

Question two: Discuss the specific pre-operative preparation that Mrs White will require.

25 minutes

Question three: Discuss the specific post-operative care that Mrs White will require.

25 minutes

Time allowance: **75 minutes**

Answer to question one:
Discuss the physiological changes that occur in the intestine as a result of obstruction.

In bowel obstruction, the bowel initially contracts with increased peristaltic activity and there is an increase in bowel sounds. However, if the increased peristaltic activity is unable to dislodge the obstruction, peristalsis stops and there is absence of bowel sounds. The fluid is pushed in the reverse direction resulting in vomiting.

Substances released by the affected intestinal wall cause some of the pathological changes such as hyperaemia, oedema and the luminal accumulation of fluid in the gut. The accumulation of gastrointestinal secretions (up to 8 litres) and swallowed air also results in abdominal distention. This sequestration (accumulation) of fluid in the gut and the reduced absorptive capacity of the gut is partially responsible for causing hypovolaemic shock, which left untreated can lead to multi-organ failure. The reduced perfusion increases anaerobic respiration and the patient may develop metabolic acidosis. The build up of intraluminal pressure increases the pressure in the bowel wall which in turn may increase the resistance in the capillaries in the mesenteric artery. This results in stagnation of bowel circulation causing oedema, necrosis and gangrene. There is increased bacterial growth in the stagnant fluid and leakage of this infected fluid can cause peritonitis. The consistency of the vomitus should be monitored as it may indicate the area of the intestine that may be obstructed.

Answer to question two:
Discuss the specific pre-operative preparation that Mrs White will require.

This will comprise of the physical and psychological preparation:

Specific physical preparation

- As dehydration is present, fluid and electrolyte replacement becomes vital. The nurse should ensure that the fluid is administered as prescribed and to monitor the patient to ensure that treatment is effective and that there are no complications. The central venous pressure (CVP) will be monitored to prevent fluid overload. Mrs White's blood pressure, pulse, temperature, respiration and urine output should be monitored to recognise signs of early complications such as shock.
- A nasogastric tube is inserted with the aim of decompressing the stomach in order to reduce the risk of inhalation of vomit (Butler, et al., 1991; Baker, et al., 1999) and to reduce the accumulation of fluid in the gut. This may be aspirated frequently as well as being placed on free drainage. If Mrs White is still nauseated, she should be given an antiemetic and supported when she is being sick. Tissues, a vomit bowl and a call bell should be within easy reach of the patient. An accurate fluid balance chart should be maintained. Mrs White may be distressed at the colour and smell of the vomit and she should be reassured and comforted.
- Mrs White will receive antibiotic therapy prophylactically preoperatively to reduce the risk of peritonitis.
- Mrs White will be kept 'nil by mouth' to reduce vomiting and minimise risk of inhalation, in anticipation of impending surgery. It is important that Mrs White receives adequate mouth care whilst she remains 'nil by mouth'.

Specific psychological preparation

It is imperative that Mrs White is psychologically prepared for this potentially life threatening surgery. The role of the nurse is to ensure that she receives information and explanation of the possible surgery and implications.

Answer to question three:
Discuss the specific post-operative care that Mrs White will require.

- On receiving the patient the nurse should check Mrs White's respiratory and circulatory status and oxygen saturation levels.
- Check drainage tubes for estimated blood loss and monitor fluid intake and output accurately. Intravenous infusions should be maintained until Mrs White is able to take oral fluids, this is dependant on her recovery and general progress. The naso gastric tube will remain on free drainage until bowel function has recovered; presence of bowel sounds, bowel activity and reduced amount of naso gastric aspirate.
- Mrs White will remain 'nil by mouth' and mouth care should be provided as necessary. Mrs White should be encouraged to rinse her mouth frequently and a suitable mouth wash should be provided.
- Post-operative pain should be managed effectively. Patient's pain should be assessed and an appropriate analgesic administered. The patient's response should be monitored and the drug titrated to achieve a therapeutic effect. Side effects should be monitored and if the patient is nauseated, an anti emetic should be given (Tate & Cook, 1996a, b). Mrs White should be provided with basic comfort measures and assisted to relax.
- The abdominal wound should be checked for haemorrhage and observed for clinical manifestations of infection: redness, swelling, tenderness, warmth, any discharge from the wound and pyrexia. Sutures should be removed after healing has taken place.
- Patients having abdominal surgery often avoid movement for fear of pain. Mrs White should be encouraged to do leg exercises and ambulate as soon as possible. The patient should also be encouraged to take at least 10 deep breaths hourly to promote full aeration of the lungs. The patient should be assisted to cough in an effort to bring up any accumulated secretions in the air passages. Mrs White should be taught to splint the wound during these procedures to minimise pain.
- Nutritional support is an important part of Mrs White's care. It is unlikely that Mrs White will be able to take fluids or diet immediately. Other methods of nutritional input should be considered until Mrs White is able to tolerate oral diet as clinically indicated.
- Ongoing, individualised psychological care will be required.

References

Baker, F., Smith, L., Stead, L. (1999) Practical procedures for nurses: inserting a nasogastric tube. Nursing Times 95(7).

Butler, J.A., Cameron, B.L., Morrow, M., Kahng, K., Tom, J. (1991) Small bowel obstruction in patients with a prior history of cancer. American Journal of Surgery 162: 624–628.

Tate, S., Cook, H. (1996a) Postoperative nausea and vomiting 1: physiology and aetiology. British Journal of Nursing 5(16): 962–973.

Tate, S., Cook, H. (1996b) Postoperative nausea and vomiting 2: management and treatment. British Journal of Nursing 5(17): 1032–1039.

Further reading

De Salvo, G.L., Gava, C., Pucciarelli, S., Lise, M. (2002) Curative surgery for obstruction from primary left colorectal carcinoma: primary or staged resection? (Cochrane Review). In: The Cochrane library, Issue 1. Oxford. Update Software.

Field, J., Bjarnason, K. (2002) Feeding patients after abdominal surgery. Nursing Standard 16(48): 41–44.

Fruer, D.J., Broadley, K.E., Sheperd, J.H., Barton, D.P.J. (2002) Surgery for the resolution of symptoms in malignant bowel obstruction and advanced gynaecological and gastrointestinal cancer (Cochrane Review). In: The Cochrane library, Issue 1. Oxford. Update Software.

Laparoscopic surgical management for an ectopic pregnancy

Abigail Moriarty

Leah Russell is a married 24-year-old primary school teacher of Afro-Caribbean background. She lives with her husband James, who is a professional artist. They live in a three bedroom detached house, both enjoy travelling and dining out with friends. Leah and James have decided to try for a family, Leah had her intrauterine device (IUD) removed by her General Practitioner (GP). Leah missed her following menstrual period and a home urine pregnancy test result was positive. A beta-human chrionic gonadotropin (HCG) blood test confirmed the pregnancy.

At 6 weeks gestation, Leah complains of severe lower abdominal pain and vaginal bleeding. She and James go to the Accident and Emergency department where she is examined by a gynaecologist who also completes an abdominal ultrasound scan. This scan showed an empty uterus, no indication of a viable foetus or intrauterine pregnancy. Leah is admitted to the gynaecology ward for an emergency laparoscopy under general anaesthetic. This showed a right fallopian tube ectopic pregnancy with rupture and bleeding requiring a right salpingectomy. Following surgery Leah returned to the ward with three abdominal laparoscope sites covered with dry dressings, an intravenous infusion (IVI) of fluids and a patient controlled analgesia (PCA) system.

Question one: Draw from memory the possible locations of an ectopic pregnancy, confirm your drawing with Figure 16.1.

15 minutes

Question two: Define what is meant by the term ectopic pregnancy.

10 minutes

Question three: Identify factors that may predispose to an ectopic pregnancy.

15 minutes

Question four: Leah had the removal of her right fallopian tube (right salpingectomy), via a laparoscope. What are the likely advantages and disadvantages of this laparoscopic procedure?

10 minutes

Question five: What psychological support may Leah and James need following her ectopic pregnancy?

10 minutes

Time allowance: **60 minutes**

Answer to question one:
Draw from memory the possible locations of an ectopic pregnancy, confirm your drawing with Figure 16.1.

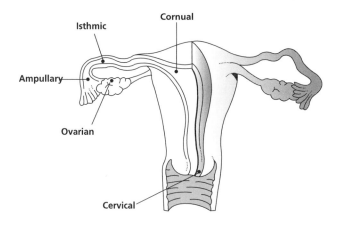

Figure 16.1: Sites of ectopic pregnancies.

Answer to question two:
Define what is meant by the term ectopic pregnancy.

An ectopic pregnancy can be defined as a gestation that implants itself outside the endometrial cavity (Moore & Hacker, 1992); it is caused by a delay in the transportation of the fertilised egg along the fallopian tube. This is an emergency situation that may present a serious hazard to Leah's health and reproductive potential. Ectopic pregnancies may be due to a combination of reasons, this will be further explored in question three. 95% of ectopic pregnancies occur in the distal ampullary region of the fallopian tube (Barclay, 2000), Leah's right fallopian tube was the location of the ectopic pregnancy.

Answer to question three:
Identify factors that may predispose to an ectopic pregnancy.

In recent years hospital admissions with ectopic pregnancy have greatly increased. In the United Kingdom there are approximately 11,000 cases per year (incidence of 11.5 per 1000 pregnancies) and resulting in four deaths (0.4 per 1000 ectopic pregnancies) (HMSO, 1998). Although a proportion of women with an ectopic pregnancy have no casual factors, several specific aspects have been implicated as contributing to the increased epidemiology.

Intrauterine device (IUD)

This contraceptive method does not cause ectopic pregnancy. In fact it effectively prevents intrauterine pregnancy but extrauterine pregnancy with an IUD is four times more likely (Ling & Stovall, 1994).

Pelvic inflammatory disease (PID)

May damage the cilia within fallopian tubes and therefore may impair and delay the transportation of the ovum to the uterus. This is particularly true of *Chlamydia trachomatis*, the major cause of PID (Hillis et al, 1995).

Tubal surgery

May have occurred for previous ectopic pregnancy, or possible reversal for sterilisations. This surgery may cause internal scarring and adhesions therefore occluding or affecting the patency of one or both of the fallopian tubes, resulting in ectopic implantation of the ovum.

Ethnic race

Ectopic pregnancy is more likely among women of Afro-Caribbean background (Barclay, 2000).

Client profiles in nursing: adult & the elderly 2

Answer to question four:
Leah had the removal of her right fallopian tube (right salpingectomy), via a laparoscope. What are the likely advantages and disadvantages of this laparoscopic procedure?

Laparoscopic procedures are considered minimal access surgery and aim to achieve the same as an open surgical operation (Yao & Tulandi, 1997). A salpingectomy would have previously been completed by performing a laparotomy (an abdominal incision), but due to medical and technical advancements in fibre optics and imaging, laparoscopic approaches are now common in gynaecology (Torrance & Serginson, 2000), although there are associated benefits and drawbacks.

Advantages

Quicker post-operative recovery and shorter hospital stay

Leah returned to the ward following her operation with a PCA system, an IVI of 1 litre of normal saline prescribed over 8 hours. Unfortunately, many patients report poor post-operative pain management while in hospital (Carr, 1997). Leah used the PCA that allowed her to activate her own administration of morphine from a preset syringe pump (but did not permit to overdose upon the morphine). Ballantyne et al (1993) suggest that a PCA can provide more effective pain relief than intramuscular injections of morphine. Leah reported her pain as slight – moderate using the verbal rating scale (Kitson, 1994) and used the PCA when in moderate pain. The PCA was removed one day post-operatively, when Leah took oral paracetamol when required.

The intravenous therapy provided Leah with hydration and electrolytes while she recovered from her anaesthetic. As Leah did not experience any post-operative nausea, she was able to resume free fluids and light diet on the first post-operative day and the IVI was discontinued.

Leah has a laparoscopic procedure the exterior wounds of which are minimal compared with a conventional salpingectomy (Olagundoye et al, 2000). Resuming ambulation, eating and drinking can commence soon after surgery, therefore reducing the time in hospital.

Decreased post-operative pain

Leah has three small abdominal incisions where the laparoscope and instruments were inserted to remove the ectopic pregnancy and damaged fallopian tube. The PCA was sufficient to manage Leah's pain but she complained of shoulder pain. This is caused by the carbon dioxide that is introduced into the peritoneum to inflate the abdominal cavity; this allows the surgeon good visualisation of the reproductive system and surrounding organs. The majority of the carbon dioxide is removed from the body at the end of the surgical procedure, any that remains within the body may push upon the diaphragm and can cause shoulder pain. This can be relieved with the PCA, a heat pad or passive exercises.

Smaller operation scar

A laparoscopic salpingectomy leaves Leah with three small incision sites a few centimetres long, which is considerably smaller than a conventional laparotomy scar.

Disadvantages

Insertion of laparoscope

A trocar is inserted into the subumbilical area, via this incision the laparoscope, telescopes and other surgical instruments are inserted into the abdominal cavity. If needed other small incisions can be made around the abdomen to accommodate other laparoscopic equipment. These incisions and the movement of the equipment within the abdomen can puncture vessels, leading to haemorrhage and peritonitis. White and Carthew (1995) state that laparoscopic surgery is changing the demands upon health care professionals, they need to adopt and develop the appropriate skills. This evolution of skills within minimal invasive surgery could reduce any complications (Mascarenhas et al, 1997).

Answer to question five:
What psychological support may Leah and James need following her ectopic pregnancy?

Miscarriage is a pregnancy loss within the first 24 weeks of gestation, which includes an ectopic pregnancy. It is a common phenomenon in gynaecology and obstetrics, Smith (1988) identified as many as one in five pregnancies result in miscarriage. Miscarriage can be associated with a variety of psychological difficulties (Nikcevic et al, 2000). Leah and James may suffer from anxiety (Thaper & Thaper, 1992), depression (Harker, 1992) and long term psychological problems following the loss of their baby (Murphy, 1998).

Counselling and advice

Many hospitals offer parents counselling following a miscarriage, where they can discuss their feelings with a nurse, doctor or counsellor. This follow up appointment would encourage Leah and James to describe the events surrounding their miscarriage and express feelings, worries and concerns. Nikcevic et al (2000) highlights that many women are concerned about their future fertility following an ectopic pregnancy and the incidence of a reoccurrence. Leah had a salpingectomy where the fallopian tube is removed therefore removing her chance of conceiving from eggs released from the right ovary, although the left ovary and tube is unaffected. Approximately 40–60% of women following an ectopic pregnancy will become pregnant again; in 10–20% of these there will be another ectopic pregnancy. Therefore Leah and James will be advised to plan future pregnancies and seek an earlier ultrasound scan to confirm an intrauterine pregnancy following her first missed menstrual period.

References

Barclay, C. (2000) Obstetrics and Gynaecology in General Practice: The Primary Care Handbook and Aide Memoire. (2nd ed.). Wiltshire: Quay Books.
Ballantyne, J.C., Carr, D.B., Chalmers, T.I., Dear, K.G.B., Anellilo, I.F. (1993) Postoperative patient controlled analgesia: meta analysis of initial randomised controlled trials. Journal of Clinical Anaesthesiology 5: 182–193.
Carr, E.C.J. (1997) Evaluating the use of a pain assessment tool and care plan – a pilot study. Journal of Advanced Nursing 26(6): 1073–1079.
Harker, L. (1992) Emotional well being following miscarriage. Journal of Obstetrics and Gynaecology 13: 262–265.
Hillis, S.D., Nakanashinma, A., Amsterdam, L. et al (1995) The impact of a comprehensive Chlamydia prevention programme in Wisconsin. Family Planning Perspectives 27: 108–111.
HMSO (1998) Why women die. Report on confidential enquiries into maternal deaths. Norwich: HMSO.
Kitson, A. (1994) Postoperative pain management: a literature review. Journal of Clinical Nursing 70: 440–442.
Ling, F.W., Stovall, T.G. (1994) Advances in Obstetrics and Gynaecology. Chicago: Mosby.
Mascarenhas, L., Williamson, J., Smith, S. (1997) The changing face of ectopic pregnancy. British Medical Journal 315: 7101–7141.

Moore, J.G., Hacker, N.F. (1992) Essentials of Gynaecology and Obstetrics. (2nd ed.). Pennsylvania: WB Saunders.

Murphy, F.A. (1998) The experience of early miscarriage from a male perspective. Journal of Clinical Nursing 7: 325–332.

Nikcevic, A.V., Kuczmieiczyk, A.R., Tunkel, S.A., Nicolaides, K.H. (2000) Distress after miscarriage: relation to the knowledge of the cause of pregnancy loss and coping style. Journal of Reproductive and Infant Psychology 18(4): 339–343.

Olagundoye, V., Adeghe, J., Guirguis, M., Cox, C., Murphy, D. (2000) Laproscopic surgical management of ectopic pregnancy: a district general hospital experience. Journal of Obstetrics and Gynaecology 20: 620–623.

Smith, N.C. (1988) Epidemiology of miscarriage. Contemporary Review of Obstetrics and Gynaecology 43: 43–48.

Thaper, A.K., Thaper, A. (1992) Psychological sequelae of miscarriage: a controlled study using the general health questionnaire and hospital anxiety and depression scale. British Journal of General Practice 42: 94–96.

Torrance, C., Serginson, E. (2000) Surgical Nursing. Edinburgh: Bailliere Tindall.

White, J., Carthew, L. (1995) The hazards of minimal access surgery. Surgical Nursing 8(3): 9–12.

Yao, M., Tulandi, T. (1997) Current status of surgical and non-surgical management of ectopic pregnancy. Fertility Sterilisation 67: 421–433.

Further reading

Cushieri, A. (1993) Ergonomics of minimal access surgery. Surgery 11(10): 526–528.

Hall, F.A. (1994) Minimal Access for Nurses and Technicians. Oxford: Radcliffe Medical Press Ltd.

Herkes, B. (2002) A bereavement counselling service for parents. British Journal of Midwifery 10(2): 79–82.

Jolley, S. (2001) Managing post-operative nausea and vomiting. Nursing Standard 15(40): 47–52.

Useful addresses

Miscarriage Association
Claydon Hospital
Northgate
Wakefield
WF1 3JS

The Ectopic Pregnancy Trust
Maternity Unit,
Hillingdon Hospital,
Pield Health Road,
Uxbridge,
Middlesex
UB8 3NN

Head injury

Danny Pertab

Matt Taylor is an 18-year-old undergraduate studying science at a local university. He is described as a friendly lad with an outgoing personality. Matt enjoys an active sports life and his pastimes include soccer, swimming and riding his motorbike.

At the end of the last semester, he was returning to his hometown on his motorbike. Due to the foggy condition, visibility was rather poor. The road condition was icy and slippery and being a Friday evening traffic on the road was heavy. At a roundabout Matt skidded and fell off his bike. Other drivers stopped to help Matt and soon the traffic came to a standstill.

Matt suffered temporary loss of consciousness, bruising to the forehead and multiple minor grazes to limbs. He soon regained consciousness but complained of dizziness and headache. He received first aid from other drivers whilst waiting for the ambulance. He was subsequently taken to the local Accident & Emergency Department, where he was examined and kept in the observation ward overnight. The following morning, the duty casualty officer checked Matt's condition and discharged him as his parents agreed to look after him. He was given specific information both in writing and verbal forms to report signs of adverse change. His parents were instructed, in the unlikely event that his condition deteriorates, he must be brought back to the casualty department immediately.

Question one: Define the nature of head injury that Matt has sustained.

15 minutes

Question two: Identify the main reason for admitting Matt to the hospital and discuss the significance of the clinical observations he will require.

30 minutes

Question three: What are the nurse's main responsibilities in caring for Matt in the first 24 hours?

15 minutes

Time allowance: **60 minutes**

Answer to question one:
Define the nature of head injury that Matt has sustained.

'Head injuries' cover a wide spectrum of injuries, involving the skull and the cranial content. It may include minor bruising to the head, scalp lacerations and to the more severe debilitating and even fatal brain damage. Head injuries may also be associated with facial injuries, neck injuries and injuries involving other parts of the body. The majority of head injuries are caused by road traffic accidents, falls and assaults, but the incidence for each cause vary according to age group (Currie et al, 2000). Falls and domestic accidents predominate in the elderly age group but assaults and industrial injuries are more common in younger age groups.

Matt sustained superficial bruising to the forehead, momentary loss of consciousness attributable to temporary dysfunction (concussion). He continued to complain of dizziness and severe headache, which could indicate a more serious underlying brain injury.

Answer to question two:
Identify the main reason for admitting Matt to the hospital and discuss the significance of the clinical observations he will require.

Hospital admission would be necessary if any of the following are present: alterations in the level of consciousness, post traumatic epileptic fit, focal neurological signs (double vision), clinical or radiological evidence of skull fracture, severe headache and vomiting, leakage of cerebrospinal fluid (CSF) from the nose or ears, extensive scalp laceration, inadequate supervision at home (Moulton & Yates, 1999).

Matt is admitted for overnight observation as a precautionary measure to observe his condition closely, detecting any early signs of deterioration and promptly instigating the necessary course of action.

Concussion, prolonged dizziness and confusion may be associated with problems like severe contusion (severe bruising of the brain), torn blood vessels and intracranial haemorrhage. Two fifths of those losing consciousness following head injuries developed raised intracranial pressure (Odell, 1996).

Frequent neurological observation and measurement of vital signs will help to recognise these complications and will be undertaken as clinically indicated. A neurological assessment tool such as the Glasgow Coma Scale (GCS) (Figure 17.1) helps to gather information more objectively on the patient's

	Score	Code
Eye opening response		
Spontaneously	4	**C** = Eyes closed by welling
To speech	3	
To pain	2	
None	1	
Best verbal response		
Orientated	5	**T** = Endotracheal tube or
Confused	4	tracheostomy
Inappropriate words	3	
Incomprehensible sounds	2	
No response	1	
Best motor response		
Obeys simple commands	6	Usually record the best arm
Localises to pain	5	movement (most people
Flexes limbs to pain	4	are right handed)
Flexes abnormally to pain	3	
Extends limbs to pain	2	
No response	1	
Total	15	

Figure 17.1: Glasgow Coma Scale (adapted from Currie et al, 2000).

conscious level, sensory and motor responses. The responses are scored on a scale of 3–15; designed to measure arousal, awareness and activity (Dawson, 2000). GCS is the most important development in the management of head injury as it makes it possible to recognise changes in consciousness reflecting recovery or deterioration (Currie et al, 2000).

Checking pupil sizes and their reaction to light provides vital information about the central nervous system. Normally, pupils should be round, equal in size and measure between 2 and 5 mm (Muxlow, 2000). Changes in pupil size and reaction to light may suggest compression of the oculomotor nerve (3rd cranial nerve). A non-reacting or dilated pupil is evidence of oculomotor nerve compression particularly when associated with diminished level of consciousness (Walsh & Kent, 2001). Non-reacting and dilated pupils associated with head injuries are late signs of complication that will develop after a fall in the level of consciousness (Walsh & Kent, 2001).

Head injuries may also affect blood pressure, pulse, respiration and temperature regulation. Hypertension with bradycardia implies raised intracranial pressure, but this sign is not always present and is a very late sign of intracranial hypertension (Sinclair, 1991). Hypotension is very rarely attributed to head injury itself, but if present, it is likely to suggest the possibility of blood loss (Currie et al, 2000) and spinal cord injury. Hyperthermia may indicate a disturbance of the hypothalamus in regulating body temperature. Immediately on admission Matt may be hypothermic due to prolonged exposure in a cold environment prior to arrival at the hospital. An accurate baseline temperature is therefore required (Walsh & Kent, 2001).

Increase in the output of dilute urine may suggest impaired tubular re-absorption in the kidneys. This may be a sign of impaired antidiuretic hormone (vasopressin) secretion from the posterior pituitary gland in the brain.

Combined with vital signs observation, neurological assessment using the GCS provides a comprehensive and objective picture of the patient's condition. It may assist in the early detection of neurological and systemic complications. Any significant change in neurological observations and vital functions must be reported immediately. The signs to be immediately reported to the medical staff include deteriorating conscious level, focal signs such as limb weakness, changes in the shapes, sizes and reaction of both pupils to direct stimulation to light, convulsive activities, nausea and vomiting, alteration in vital signs like respiration, blood pressure, temperature and pulse rate; leaks from the nose and ear (possibly loss of CSF) are indicative of open fracture/s at the base of the skull.

Answer to question three:
What are the nurse's main responsibilities in caring for Matt in the first 24 hours?

The nurse's responsibilities, at this stage of Matt's admission includes: maintaining his safety, bedrest and general comfort, frequent observation of vital functions (consciousness, airway, breathing and circulation) and neurological status, protection of cervical spine, early detection of any ensuing complications and giving relevant information to reassure him of his safety, sense of control and best interest as well as supporting during investigations such as skull X-ray or computerised tomography.

Matt's nursing care will include rest. As a conscious patient he is nursed in a position most comfortable to him; although it may be desirable to slightly elevate the head of the bed (no more than 30°) as gravity promotes venous drainage via the jugular and vertebral veins (Muxlow, 2000) and easing pressure within the cranial cavity. He should be located in a quiet and dimly lit room to reduce irritability, photophobia and undue interference. Other aspects of care may consist of oxygen therapy to ease possible hypoxia, effective communication to orientate him to the environment thus minimising possible confusion. Pain relief for headache will be administered (if there are no contra indications), treatment of nausea if it arises, nutritional and fluid intakes, and general hygiene to promote personal comfort are integral to the total package of optimum care. Voiding of urine must be noted to eliminate the risk of bladder distension and its associated discomfort due to immobility. Gentle deep breathing exercise and limb movement must be encouraged to preserve pulmonary functions, muscle tone and to prevent complications of immobility. Such nursing measures will enhance the chances of successful rehabilitation and early return to normality.

Discharge planning will include giving Matt and his parents verbal and written information about his condition and to report any significant changes to Accident and Emergency staff.

References

Currie, D.E., Ritchie, E., Stott, S. (2000) The Management of Head Injuries: A Practical Guide for The Emergency Room. (2nd ed.). Oxford: Oxford University Press.

Dawson, D. (2000) Neurological care. In: Shepherd, M., Wright, S. (2000) (Eds) Principles and Practice of High dependency Nursing. Edinburgh: Bailliere Tindall in Association with The Royal College of Nursing.

Moulton, C., Yates, D. (1999) Head injuries: Lectures on Emergency Medicine. (2nd ed.). Oxford: Blackwell Science.

Muxlow, J. (2000) Caring for the neurologic system. In: Bassett, C., Makin, L. (2000) (Eds) Caring for seriously ill patients. London: Arnold Publishers.

Odell, M. (1996) 'Intracranial pressure monitoring, nursing in a district general hospital'. Nursing in Critical Care 1(5): 245–247.

Sinclair, M. (1991) Nursing the Neurological Patient. Oxford: Butterworth-Heinmann.

Walsh, M., Kent, A. (2001) Accident & Emergency Nursing. (4th ed.). Oxford: Butterworth-Heinmann.

Further reading

Woodrow, P. (2000) Neurological monitoring and intracranial hypertension. Intensive Care Nursing: A Framework for Practice. London: Routledge: Taylor & Francis Group.

Post-operative pain

Sam Parboteeah

Mr Cheng, a 66-year-old man has returned from surgery having had resection of the large bowel for cancer. He is conscious and responding to verbal commands.

He has a good command of English language. He lives with his wife and five children; his wife speaks limited English but the children speak fluently and are able to translate information for her. He runs a Chinese food outlet and all the family help with the business.

His hydration is being maintained intravenously and he is 'nil by mouth'. A visual check of the abdomen shows a transverse surgical incision covered with a surgical dressing. A drain and a urinary catheter are in situ.

An intravenous infusion of morphine is being administered at the rate of 2 mg per hour via a continuous infusion pump. His observations are as follows: blood pressure 140/90 mmHg; pulse 120 beats per minute; respiration rate at 18 breaths per minute and a temperature of 37°C.

After settling Mr Cheng in bed the nurse asked if he had any pain. He grimaced and replied that he was in a 'lot of pain'.

Question one: Discuss the importance of pain assessment in the management of Mr Cheng's pain.

20 minutes

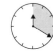

Question two: What are the possible physiological consequences of pain in the post surgical patient?

20 minutes

Question three: Describe how Mr Cheng's pain may be brought under control.

20 minutes

Time allowance: **60 minutes**

Answer to question one:
Discuss the importance of pain assessment in the management of Mr Cheng's pain.

Pain assessment

Assessing pain is an integral part of the management of pain and is a major nursing activity. As a result of assessment, pain can be identified and effective treatment started. Pain assessment is important for a number of reasons:

1. avoids nurses making erroneous assumption about the cause and extent of patient's pain.
2. prevents physical and psychological complications arising from ineffective pain management.
3. accurate reporting of pain can have a significant impact on decisions made by nurses and doctors.

Methods of assessing pain

At present, there is no objective measure that accurately evaluates the patient's pain. Hence Mr Cheng's description and quantification of the experience of pain is by far the most direct method of measuring pain and is based on the patient's assessment of the pain rather than assessment made by nurses.

Many different pain assessment tools are now available and these can be used to gather information about the quality of pain, the location and the intensity of the pain. The qualitative nature of the pain is described through the use of adjectives such as sharp, burning and stabbing. The location is the abdominal surgical wound but other locations such as pressure areas or arthritic pain should be taken into account. Pain intensity is the magnitude of the pain sensation and is the most frequently assessed dimension of pain. Caunt (1992) suggests that post-operative pain requires a short assessment in order to minimise the disturbance to the recovering patient. Many tools have been designed to measure the magnitude of pain such as the category scales (Fig. 18.1 and 18.2).

An advantage of the category scale for a post-operative patient is the ease in using it in clinical practice as illustrated in the scenario.

Mild	Moderate	Severe

Figure 18.1: A verbal descriptor scale.

0 - - - - - - - - - - - - - - - -10
No pain   Severe pain

Figure 18.2: A visual analogue scale.

Pain also activates a whole series of physiological responses of the autonomic nervous system such as hypertension, tachycardia, dilated pupils, tachypnoea, changes in colour of skin, perspiration, and reduced mental alertness. The relationship between pain and physiological responses should continue to be part of the assessment process especially in the post-operative patient where the ability to verbalise may be impaired by the effects of anaesthetic drugs.

Assessing affective and cognitive dimensions prior to surgery (in preassessment clinics) can provide vital information to the nurse in managing post-operative pain. For example, previous experiences of surgery can influence how the patient perceives how their pain will be managed.

Pain assessment is a dynamic process; initially a detailed assessment should be carried out, however, reassessment may require fewer dimensions to be assessed. The timing of the follow up is important and should correspond to the onset, peak effect and dissipation time of the drug in use.

Answer to question two:
What are the possible physiological consequences of pain in the post surgical patient?

Pain is an essential component of normal body function. It exists for human survival acting as a warning signal to avoid further injury. However, it is open to question whether pain following surgery to body tissues serves a useful purpose. Initially, it may appear to promote rest and healing because it inhibits the patient's movement. Anticipation and sensation of pain may predispose to psychological and physical development of complications.

- Anticipation of pain raises levels of anxiety and fear which leads to a rise in 17-hydroxycorticosteroid which decreases resistance to infection and slows wound healing.
- The physical sensation of pain following abdominal surgery as is the case with Mr Cheng is not only distressing but also inhibits adequate pulmonary ventilation and limits movement. Inadequate lung expansion and immobility are known to predispose to complications such as deep vein thrombosis, pneumonia and prolonged paralytic ileus.
- An increase in the sympathetic system output results in an outpouring of epinephrine (adrenaline) which results in an increase in blood pressure, increase in pulse rate and pulse pressure, rapid and irregular respirations and an increase in perspiration. These physiological changes may cause further complications in patients who have existing cardiac disease such as angina.
- The patient may also be restless and there may be an increase in muscle tension.

Answer to question three:
Describe how Mr Cheng's pain may be brought under control.

Despite recent advances in pain control over the last decade, many patients in hospitals continue to suffer unrelieved pain and up to three quarters of patients experience moderate to severe pain whilst in hospital (Royal College of Surgeons and College of Anaesthetists, 1990). McCaffery's (1979) definition of pain highlights the subjectivity of the pain experience by suggesting that 'pain is whatever the experiencing person says it is and exists whenever they say it does'. Post-operative nursing interventions aimed at making the patient comfortable and reducing his pain requires an accurate assessment of Mr Cheng's pain. It is also important to distinguish between surgical pain and any other type of pain.

Since Mr Cheng is reporting having 'a lot of pain', urgent action is required to provide pain relief. Nursing intervention will therefore include:

- Giving analgesics as prescribed to control the pain. The development of newer methods of analgesia administration such as patient-controlled analgesia (PCA), continuous intravenous infusion or epidural infusion of opiates and local anaesthetics has provided the opportunity for greater pain relief and avoids some of the problems associated with traditional intramuscular narcotic administration. In Mr Cheng's case, the intravenous infusion of morphine should be increased to a higher rate and if pain still persists an additional drug may be administered. There are many other non-pharmacologic interventions which have been used effectively in the management of pain. These include distraction, relaxation, touch, transcutaneous nerve stimulation (TENS), biofeedback, verbal support, music, massage, aromatherapy, acupuncture and reflexology. The nurse should explore with Mr Cheng any preference he may have as it is important for the patient to be fully involved in the regimen.
- During the post-operative period, the nature of the pain experienced and the patient's pain threshold and tolerance are important factors. Pain threshold and tolerance vary depending on the patient's age, gender, race, personality, culture, learning environment and uncertainty about outcome. Thus, Mr Cheng should be nursed in a more relaxed environment and information given as well as the reduction of noxious stimuli which can aggravate the pain sensation.
- Provide basic comfort measures such as proper temperature, ventilation, and visitors. Provide reassurance that the discomfort is temporary and that medication will aid in pain reduction.
- Assist patients in maintaining a positive attitude (Nettina, 1996).
- If the nurse is unable to control Mr Cheng's pain effectively, then medical staff/pain team should be contacted for help at the earliest opportunity to prevent any further delay in Mr Cheng receiving treatment.

References

Caunt, H. (1992) Reducing the psychological impact of post-operative pain. British Journal of Nursing 1: 23.

McCaffery, M. (1979) Nursing Management of the Patient with Pain. Philadelphia: Lippincott.

Nettina, S.M. (1996) The Lippincott Manual of Nursing Practice. (6th ed.). Philadelphia: Lippincott.

Royal College of Surgeons of England and College of Anaesthetists (1990) Commission on the provision of surgical services. Report of the Working Party on Pain after Surgery Royal College of Surgeons and College of Anaesthetists, London.

Further reading

Thomas, T., Robinson, C., Champion, D., McKell, M., Pell, M. (1998) Prediction and assessment of the severity of post operative pain and of satisfaction with management. Pain 75: 177–185.

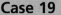

Pneumothorax

Kim Leong

Mr Alex Jones is a 60-year-old retired teacher. He lives with his 58-year-old wife in a semi-detached house. They have three daughters who all live locally. They have six grandchildren between the ages of 12 and 16 years. The grandchildren visit their grandfather and grandmother most weekends, and sometimes help them with cleaning, gardening and cooking.

Mr Jones likes to play golf at the local golf club every Tuesday morning. He thoroughly enjoys meeting up with his retired friends.

One morning, as he was preparing to go and play golf, he fell outside his house tightly clutching his chest. His next door neighbour, found him lying on the front porch. He immediately rang the emergency ambulance.

On admission to hospital he was found to be hyperventilating, cyanosed and anxious. His vital signs were recorded as: temperature 37.6°C, pulse 120 beats per minute, respiratory rate 24 per minute and blood pressure 140/90 mmHg. He was also experiencing severe chest pain.

Question one: What is a pneumothorax?

5 minutes

Question two: What are the underlining pathophysiological changes and the clinical features that Mr Jones may exhibit?

15 minutes

Question three: Discuss the medical treatment and specific nursing care that Mr Jones may receive.

20 minutes

Question four: Discuss how the under water seal drain is set up and explain how it works.

20 minutes

Time allowance: **60 minutes**

Client profiles in nursing: adult & the elderly 2

Answer to question one:
What is a pneumothorax?

The lungs are attached to the thoracic cage by serous membranes known as the pleurae (Hinchliff et al, 1996). There are two pleural membranes. The inner layer or visceral pleura covers the inner surface of each lung and is continuous with the outer layer or parietal pleura, which is closely attached to the outer surface of the thoracic cavity. If this pleura is broken by a spontaneous intra-pulmonary air leak, during surgery or by a stab wound, air will then escape from the injured lung into the pleural cavity and will then abolish the negative intrapleural pressure. This is called pneumothorax (Fig. 19.1) and the affected lung collapses resulting in seriously impaired gaseous exchange (Paradisco, 1999). 'Pneum' comes from the Greek word 'pneumatos', meaning breath, air, gas and lung; here it is used to mean air. Hence, pneumothorax means air in the thorax (Hutton, 1993).

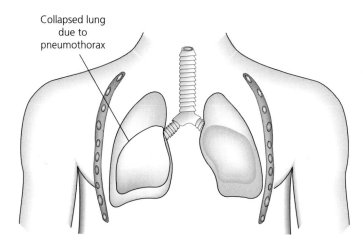

Collapsed lung
due to
pneumothorax

Figure 19.1: Partially collapsed lung with air (pneumothorax) between the pleura.

Answer to question two:
What are the underlining pathophysiological changes and the clinical features that Mr Jones may exhibit?

Each time Mr Jones inhales, more air is accumulated in the pleural cavity and as a consequence, air pressure rises and this causes the affected lung to collapse. The rising pressure within the pleural cavity of the affected lung can sometimes displace the heart and mediastinum to the unaffected side. If treatment is not carried out quickly the function of the heart will be impaired.

There is diminished or absent breath sounds on the affected lung. There is also decreased movement of the affected lung on inspiration. Since there is only one functioning lung, Mr Jones will experience difficulty in breathing, cyanosis, tachycardia and chest pain.

Answer to question three:
Discuss the medical treatment and specific nursing care that Mr Jones may receive.

A portable chest X-ray usually confirms the diagnosis. Treatment is aimed at restoring the lung to its original size and function as quickly as possible. This is usually achieved by the insertion of an under water seal drain (UWSD) into the pleural space (Fig. 19.2). The primary objective of the under water seal drain is to drain air and excess fluid and also prevent the re-entry of air into the pleural cavity. Drainage also depends on gravity and the mechanism of respiration. Sometimes gentle suction is prescribed to aid drainage, in which case a vacuum pump may be attached to the outlet tube.

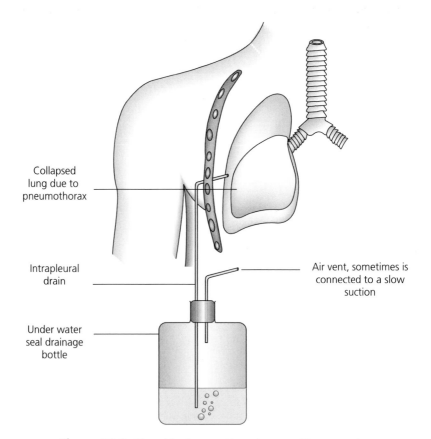

Collapsed lung due to pneumothorax

Intrapleural drain

Air vent, sometimes is connected to a slow suction

Under water seal drainage bottle

Figure 19.2: Blood between the pleura with an under water seal drainage system (a single bottle).

Respiratory support

The nurse should monitor vital signs such as blood pressure and pulse so that any internal haemorrhage can be detected and rectified immediately. Pulse oximetry should also be monitored to detect any signs of poor oxygen saturation that may interfere with Mr Jones' bodily functions. Oxygen can be prescribed and administered as clinically indicated. To promote lung expansion Alex should be nursed sitting upright or in a comfortable position.

Since there is direct contact into the pleural cavity, there is an obvious risk of the introduction of microorganisms that may cause infections. Therefore the nurse must maintain the strictest aseptic method when changing the UWSD bottles. Mr Jones must be offered appropriate analgesia (Abrams, 2001) especially before chest physiotherapy is carried out. Chest physiotherapy is carried out in order to prevent any potential chest infections (Walsh, 1997).

An airtight dressing should be applied with firm pressure after the removal of the intrapleural drain. A check chest X-ray is then carried out to determine if the affected lung has expanded to its original size.

Answer to question four:
Discuss how the under water seal drain is set up and explain how it works.

The volume of sterile water placed in the UWSD bottle should be a pre-set amount and the same volume should be used consistently throughout the hospital to prevent any potential confusion among staff. The amount should be enough to submerge the drainage tube by 2.5 cm and in most systems the amount of sterile water used is 500 millilitres. The water level is very carefully checked before the system is connected to the patient.

A suture is put in place with strong adhesive in order to prevent the intrapleural tube from accidentally becoming disconnected. The connections between the intrapleural drain and the down pipe should also be secured with transparent adhesive so that inspection can be made if needed. The junction between the down pipe and the collection bottle should similarly be sealed and secured with clear adhesive. The pleural tubing should be secured, to ensure there is no kinking, looping, twisting or pressure on the tubing and thus prevent malfunction.

Two pairs of chest drain clamps must be placed at hand near Mr Jones' bed. These clamps would be used if there was disconnection or breakage to the UWSD bottle. In such cases, the pleural tubing must be clamped off immediately to avoid renewed pneumothorax and consequently collapse of the lung. Two clamps should also be applied to the tubing when the UWSD bottle needs changing.

When mobilising, Mr Jones should be advised not to lift the UWSD bottle higher than his chest as it will cause the water from the bottle to siphon into the chest cavity.

The nurse must observe for any oscillation in the tubing. The presence of oscillation and bubbles signifies that the air is being removed from the pleural cavity. If there is no sign of the above it may mean that the tube is kinked or blocked.

The amount of drainage and its composition should be measured and recorded regularly.

References

Abrams, A.C. (2001) Clinical Drug Therapy: Rationales for Nursing Practice. New York: Lippincott.
Hinchliff, S.M., Montague, S.E., Watson, R. (1996) Physiology for Nursing Practice. (2nd ed.). London: Bailliere Tindall.
Hutton, A.R. (1993) An introduction to Medical Terminology: A Self-Teaching Package. London: Churchill Livingstone.
Paradisco, C. (1999) Lippincott's Review Series: The Ideal Study Aid. Here's Why.... Pathophysiology. (2nd ed.). New York: Lippincott.
Walsh, M. (1997) Watson's Clinical Nursing & Related Science. (5th ed.). London: Bailliere Tindall.

Blood transfusion

Penny Tremayne

Glenda Matthews is a 45-year-old business woman who lives with her partner Gary a mechanical engineer. They live in a converted barn on the outskirts of a market town. Gary's three children from a previous marriage visit every other weekend.

Glenda and Gary enjoy travelling both in the United Kingdom and around the world. Recently they have returned from a month in Australia and soon plan a safari trip to Kenya. They eat out frequently, about twice a week, their favourite being Thai food.

Glenda smokes 20 cigarettes a day and most evenings they consume a bottle of wine. Glenda has been feeling burning type pains in her stomach, the pain often exacerbating some 2–3 hours after eating and becoming increasingly more persistent. No amount of indigestion tablets or analgesics seem to relieve it. One day, whilst preparing the evening meal Glenda suddenly vomits a large amount of 'coffee ground' vomitus, this is accompanied by severe abdominal pain and she looks pale, clammy and is shaking. Gary calls for the ambulance immediately. Glenda is admitted to Maple Ward where half hourly observations of blood pressure, pulse and respiratory rate are recorded and monitored. A urinary catheter is inserted and the hourly urine output is in excess of 30 millilitres an hour. A central line is inserted to monitor central venous pressure and a cannula inserted into the back of her left hand and 500 millilitres of plasma protein substitute is infused.

Blood is taken from Glenda for cross-matching and rhesus D compatibility, and full blood count including haemoglobin concentration. The result of the haemoglobin concentration is 7.4 g/dl; Glenda is prescribed a blood transfusion of four units of whole blood. Meanwhile an urgent endoscopy is hastily arranged to identify the possible causes of bleeding.

Question one: Discuss the ward involvement and preparations that are necessary prior to the transfusion of blood.

25 minutes

Question two: Explain the principles of care that Glenda will require throughout the blood transfusion.

20 minutes

Question three: Briefly describe the possible adverse reactions of a blood transfusion.

15 minutes

Time allowance: **60 minutes**

Answer to question one:
Discuss the ward involvement and preparations that are necessary prior to the transfusion of blood.

There are a number of checks to consider prior to commencing Glenda's blood transfusion. However, it can be suggested that the single most important check is to ensure that the local policy/protocol is strictly applied to all aspects of blood transfusion administration. Another fairly obvious check is to ensure that the blood transfusion has actually been prescribed (Fig. 20.1) and that Glenda has an awareness of what is proposed and why. The next check is related to the person who takes the blood sample for ABO/rhesus D testing and cross matching. Asher et al (2002) and the British Committee for Standards in Haematology (BCSH, 1999) highlight that the person should check Glenda's full name, gender, date of birth, identification number. This should then be verified verbally by Glenda, by details on Glenda's wristband and by details on her blood request form. Prior labelling of a sample bottle should always be avoided (BCSH, 1999). The person collecting blood from the blood storage bank should take some patient documentation which contains patient details alongside details of what is to be collected (McKenna, 2000). Then the unit of blood should be cross checked with documentation from the ward and the cross-match/compatibility label (Atterbury, 2001a). Every unit of blood that is withdrawn from the refrigerator should be documented according to local policy/protocol. Blood should be removed from the blood storage bank no more than 30 minutes before administration, as any longer would facilitate the risk of bacterial growth in the blood. The patency of Glenda's intravenous cannula should be checked as well as security, and Atterbury (2001a) suggests that a 20 gauge cannula is appropriate. Before immediate administration of the blood transfusion another vital check has to be undertaken and this will often vary countrywide according to local protocol. The BCSH (1999) have recommended that it is appropriate for one registered nurse to be responsible to perform the final checking procedure. This final check should always be performed by the bedside of the patient. This check will include:

- Confirmation of verbal consent again.
- Appropriate equipment to commence transfusion namely: a drip stand, a blood giving set which includes a filter to trap any debris, gloves and possibly a pump, observation charts.
- The checking of baseline observations: temperature, pulse, respiration, blood pressure and commence fluid balance chart.
- Positive identification of the patient if able verbally and by wristband detailing, name, identification number, date of birth.
- Patient details need to be checked and be identical, this includes: the wristband, the blood transfusion compatibility label (blood group, blood product and the blood unit number), the compatibility label attached to the blood pack (blood group, blood product and the blood unit number), the prescription chart and the medical notes.
- The expiry date of that unit of blood.

DOCTOR PRESCRIBING A BLOOD COMPONENT MUST GO THROUGH THE FOLLOWING CHECKLIST. IF THE RESPONSE TO ANY OF THE FOLLOWING IS YES, THE PATIENT MUST RECEIVE IRRADIATED CELLULAR BLOOD COMPONENTS:-

1. Allograft recipient. Yes/No
2. Autograft recipient (NO TBI) <3 months post transplant. Yes/No
3. Autograft recipient (TBI) <6 months post transplant. Yes/No
4. Hodgkin's disease. Yes/No
5. Due for bone marrow/Peripheral blood harvest in next 7 days. Yes/No
6. Currently on or has at any time received Fludarabine/Cladrabine/Deoxycofromycin/Campath. Yes/No
7. Due to receive HLA matched platelets. Yes/No

8. Due to receive intrauterine transfusion. Yes/No
9. Due to receive red cell exchange transfusion during first 6 months of life. Yes/No
10. Platelet/red cell transfusion for a child under 6 months of age who has previously received an intrauterine transfusion. Yes/No
11. Suspected or confirmed congenital cellular Immunodeficiency state. Yes/No

HOSPITAL NO. ....
SURNAME ....
FORENAMES ....
DOB ....
ADDRESS ....

DATE	BLOOD COMPONENT	DOSE/ VOLUME	*STATE IF CMV NEG./ IRRADIATED/ HLA MATCHED OR NOT APPLICABLE	RATE OF INFUSION	OTHER SPECIFIC INSTRUCTIONS (E.G. IF A DIURETIC IS REQUIRED)	DR'S SIG. & INITIALS	CHECKED BY SIG. & INITIALS	ADMIN SIG. & INITIALS	Time Started	Time Completed	PRE T	PRE P	PRE B/P	20 MIN T	20 MIN P	20 MIN B/P	60 MIN T	60 MIN P	60 MIN B/P
A																			
		UNIT BAR CODE NUMBER:																	
B																			
		UNIT BAR CODE NUMBER:																	
C																			
		UNIT BAR CODE NUMBER:																	
D																			
		UNIT BAR CODE NUMBER:																	
E																			
		UNIT BAR CODE NUMBER:																	
F																			
		UNIT BAR CODE NUMBER:																	
G																			
		UNIT BAR CODE NUMBER:																	

MANDATORY

THIS COLUMN IS MANDATORY. THE CLINICAL STAFF RESPONSIBLE FOR ADMINISTERING BLOOD COMPONENTS SHOULD CHECK THAT A DOCTOR HAS COMPLETED THIS COLUMN PRIOR TO COMMENCING TRANSFUSION.

Figure 20.1: Blood component prescription and administration chart.

- A visual check of the integrity of the blood: air bubbles, colour or clotting of blood.
- Signature of those who have undertaken the check must be recorded on the compatibility sheet and dated. The prescription of the blood transfusion must also be dated, timed and signed.

BCSH (1999) and Bradbury and Cruickshank (2000)

Answer to question two:
Explain the principles of care that Glenda will require throughout the blood transfusion.

Once again, it must be reiterated that local protocol should be applied in the care of Glenda throughout her blood transfusion. General principles will include the aseptic handling of the blood transfusion throughout the procedure. Particular attention must be paid to the cannula in Glenda's left hand which should have a clear dressing to secure it and frequent observation of the area for signs of redness, inflammation or extravasation. The blood should be transfused at the appropriate rate. A calculation will take into account the drops per millilitre and volume of the blood to be transfused. More increasingly blood is being transfused via pumps. It is vital that the nurse has a good knowledge and understanding of how the pump works and that the pump is suitable, the BCSH (1999) highlighting that red cells can be damaged by electronic infusion pumps. The calculation of the blood transfusion rate is important because lengthy delays will result in increased bacterial growth and the leakage of potassium from donor cells (McClelland, 2001). The usual duration is 2–3 hours (BCSH, 1999). Recordings of temperature, pulse rate, respiratory rate and blood pressure will be recorded when each unit of blood is commenced and completed. These vital signs should be measured 15 minutes after the commencement of each unit of blood. A change in these observations may indicate an adverse reaction so a member of medical staff should be alerted as soon as possible, and the transfusion stopped. One of the most important principles is to observe Glenda: does she have any signs of discomfort, pain, rash, flushing, breathing problems? Once again if she does, the blood transfusion should be ceased and medical staff informed. A fluid balance chart should be maintained and the colour and amount of urine monitored. Glenda may require medication whilst blood is being transfused; this should be administered as per local protocol. Glenda will also require assistance with activities of living to ensure that she has a call bell close to hand and that she is in an easily observable position. Glenda may well be anxious, so explain to her what is going on, giving her every reassurance possible. A leaflet has been prepared for The National Health Service about 'Receiving a Blood Transfusion'. Care should be meticulously noted within Glenda's nursing documentation.

Answer to question three:
Briefly describe the possible adverse reactions of a blood transfusion.

There are a number of adverse reactions that can occur as a consequence of a blood transfusion:

- Pulmonary oedema as a result of cardiac overload. The patient will be breathless, and coughing and, as in this case, there will be a rise in the central venous pressure recording. Patients can be prescribed a diuretic alongside the blood transfusion. The patient should be nursed sitting up and a strict fluid balance chart maintained.
- An acute haemolytic reaction is one in which there are signs of increased red cell destruction. It usually is a result of ABO mismatch and occurs generally within 15 minutes of the transfusion commencing. The patient may experience anything from mild to the most severe of symptoms including: chest pain, loin pain, breathlessness, rigors, flushing, oliguria, oozing from wounds or puncture sites, hypotension, tachycardia. Patient's airway, breathing and circulatory function will be monitored, all vital signs and urine output recorded. As Campbell (1996), Atterbury (2001b) indicate management should focus on maintaining the patient's blood pressure and renal perfusion.
- An allergic reaction as a consequence of plasma proteins in the donor's blood. The patient may present with flushing, itching, rashes, wheezing, chest tightness, urticarial hives and even laryngeal oedema. The most severe reaction could result in anaphylactic shock. Management will include the administration of oral or intravenous antihistamines, steroids and even adrenaline in the case of anaphylactoid reaction.
- Infective shock is a rare, possibly fatal reaction which is caused by bacterial contamination of the blood. The patient will be hypotensive and tachycardic (Atterbury, 2001b).

If any adverse reaction occurs then the blood transfusion should be stopped immediately, and medical staff alerted as soon as possible. It is common practice for the implicated blood pack and adjoining (or attached) equipment such as the giving set to be retained intact and complete. The giving set should be disconnected from the cannula and returned to the laboratory with the bag still connected.

Acknowledgement

John Revill, Process Manager, Department of Blood Transfusion, United Hospitals of Leicester NHS Trust for advice and permission for the figure used in this case.

References

Asher, D., Atterbury, C.L.J., Cohen, C., Jones, H., Love, E.M., Norfolk, D.R., Revill, J., Soldan, K., Todd, A., Williamson, L.M. (2002) Serious Hazards of Transfusion: Summary of annual report 2000–2001. Manchester: Shot Office.

Atterbury, C. (2001a) Practical procedures for nurses: blood transfusion – 1. Nursing Times 97(24): 45–46.

Atterbury, C. (2001b) Practical procedures for nurses: blood transfusion – 4. Nursing Times 97(28): 45–46.

Bradbury, M., Cruickshank, J. (2000) Blood transfusion: crucial steps in maintaining safe practice. British Journal of Nursing 9(1): 134–138.

British Committee for Standards in Haematology (1999) The administration of blood and blood components and the management of transfused patients. Transfusion Medicine 9: 227–238.

Campbell, J. (1996) Blood groups and transfusions. Professional Nurse 12(1): 39–44.

McClelland, D.B.L. (2001) Handbook of Transfusion Medicine. (3rd ed.). London: The Stationery Office.

McKenna, C. (2000) Blood minded. Nursing Times 96(14): 27–29.

Suggested reading

Atterbury, C. (2001) Practical procedures for nurses – blood transfusion – 2 and 3. Nursing Times 97(25 and 27): 43–44 and 45–46.

Gray, S., Murphy, M. (1999) Guidelines for administering blood and blood components. Nursing Standard 14(13–15): 36–39.

Higgins, C. (2000) The risks associated with blood and blood product transfusion. British Journal of Nursing 9(22): 2281–2290.

Todd, A., Gray, S. (1999) Transfusion hazards – room for improvement. Nursing Standard 13(36): 31–32.

Websites

Serious Hazards of Transfusion (www.shot.demon.co.uk)
The National Blood Service (www.blood.co.uk)
British Blood Transfusion Society (www.bbts.org.uk)

Leaflets

National Health Service – Receiving a Blood Transfusion – this valuable leaflet can be obtained from most hospital blood transfusion laboratories or from the National Blood Transfusion Service.

Colorectal cancer

Penny Harrison

Perry Manley, is a 50-year-old married father, with two grown up children and three grandchildren. Perry is a sales representative for a pharmaceutical firm. His area of work covers a large region. Perry often works and travels away from home for up to four nights in a week. He eats his meals in the hotel restaurants. Perry was previously a heavy smoker of forty cigarettes per day, but successfully gave up 12 months ago. He enjoys two glasses of wine with his evening meal, stating that it helps him to relax at the end of a busy working day. Perry is overweight at 95 kilograms, rarely takes exercise and weekends are spent with the family during the day, but catching up with paper work in the evenings.

Perry has been to see his General Practitioner (GP) recently with a history of altered bowel habit. Perry usually defaecates in the mornings, but recently has had some episodes of constipation and 'feeling bloated'. Twelve weeks ago Perry had an episode of diarrhoea, which at the time he attributed to ingestion of food at a restaurant that had 'upset his system'. However the diarrhoea has continued intermittently. A rectal examination, and stool sample to date have all been negative. Perry was referred to the local hospital for further tests and investigations for his diarrhoea and altered bowel habit. A flexible sigmoidoscopy was performed and the sigmoid colon was found to be normal. However a later colonoscopy has revealed that Perry has a mass in the colon. Biopsies taken reveal that the mass is malignant, but localised, being contained within the bowel wall. A surgical admission is planned for a resection of the colon and the surgeon is hopeful that a colostomy will not be required.

Exercise

Draw from memory an accurately labelled diagram of the large bowel and confirm your drawing with Figure 21.1.

Question one: Define flexible sigmoidoscopy and colonoscopy and explain why these tests would be required for Perry.

20 minutes

Question two: How can the nurse assist Perry and his family to come to terms with his diagnosis?

20 minutes

Client profiles in nursing: adult & the elderly 2

The colorectal cancer will be classed using a classification system. For colorectal cancer there are two main systems used: the Duke's Classification System and TNM Staging System (Knowles, 2002). Dependant on Perry's condition, information gained and how his colorectal cancer has been classified, chemotherapy and/or radiotherapy may be indicated prior to the surgery or postoperatively.

Lunn et al (1999) defines these adjunctive treatments as follows:

- Chemotherapy – is systemic treatment that is toxic to dividing cells and inhibits cell replication.
- Radiotherapy – is a local treatment that damages the DNA (deoxyribonucleic acid) and disrupts cell metabolism causing reproductive cell death.

Perry and his family may have no knowledge of the role of chemotherapy and radiotherapy. Alternatively, they may have anecdotal information or experience of adjunctive therapies and be fearful of perceived issues relating to these. Perry and his family require information about the types, routes of administration, duration, benefits, side effects and management of any adjunctive treatment. In consultation with the oncologist, decisions about radiotherapy and chemotherapy can be discussed fully. The nurse is ideally placed to ensure that Perry and his family understand the nature of the treatments. Tolerance of both adjunctive therapies may be greater if the patient is aware of any potential problems and how these are likely to be managed (Campbell 1999b). An example of this could be the management of nausea and vomiting associated with the administration of chemotherapy.

Campbell and Borwell (1999) argue that specialist nurses within patient settings are ideally placed to co-ordinate patient care. This is especially important where the patient has received care from a large or complex multi professional team across a variety of clinical settings. Nurse specialists offer expertise from their area of practice as well as continuity of care at a time where the patient and family may feel frightened and particularly vulnerable. This care is also based on the patient experience and health outcomes rather than the more traditional basis of medically orientated tasks.

References

Boyle, P. (1998) Some recent developments in the epidemiology of colorectal cancer. In: Bleiberg, H., Rougier, P., Wilkie, H-J. Management of Colorectal Cancer. London: Martin Dunitz.

Calman, K., Hine, D. (1995) Policy for Commissioning Cancer Services. London: The Stationery Office.

Campbell, T. (1999a) Colorectal cancer. Part 1: Epidemiology, aetiology, screening and diagnosis. Professional Nurse 14(12): 869–874.

Campbell, T. (1999b) Colorectal cancer. Part 3: Patient care. Professional Nurse 15(2): 117–121.

Campbell, T., Borwell, B. (1999) Colorectal cancer. Part 4: Specialist nurse roles. Professional Nurse 15(3): 197–200.

Department of Health (2000) National Service Framework for Cancer. London: The Stationery Office.

Howie, E., Miller, M.E.A., Murchie, M.B. (2000) Chapter 4 'The gastrointestinal system, liver and bilary tract. In: Alexander, M., Fawcett, J., Runciman, P. (2nd ed.). Nursing Practice Hospital and Home: The Adult. Edinburgh: Churchill Livingstone.

Knowles, G. (2002) The management of colorectal cancer. Nursing Standard 16(17): 47–52.

Lunn, D., Hurrell, C., Campbell, T. (1999) Colorectal cancer. Part 2: Treatment Professional Nurse 15(1): 53–55.

Nursing and Midwifery Council (2002) Code of Professional Conduct. London: NMC.

Sawyer, H. (2000) Meeting the information needs of cancer patients. Professional Nurse 15(4): 244–247.

Further reading

Bruce, L., Finlay, T. (1997) (Eds) Nursing in Gastroenterology. Edinburgh: Churchill Livingstone.

Cotton, P., Williams, C. (1996) Practical Gastrointestinal Endoscopy. (4th ed.). Oxford: Blackwell Scientific.

Sexually transmitted infections

Chris Buswell

'Come in Mr Donaldson, it's not often I see you of late. How are things now that you've moved into the sheltered accommodation flats?'

'Hello Doctor. Yes I'm fine and the new flat is just grand. It's brought me a new lease of life. I've got everything I need, even my own small kitchen, although I tend to eat out a lot with my new friends. The ladies there are very agreeable and seem to have taken me under their wings. In fact I wish I'd more time to spend with them all.'

'Good, good,' laughed Doctor Wilson, 'and what brings you here today?'

'Well it's a bit embarrassing doctor,' replied Mr Donaldson. 'I'm due to see Mary tomorrow, she's my favourite lady in the complex, but I feel that I can't.'

'Oh,' the doctor inquired, 'why ever not?'

'Well, at my age you don't expect these things to happen. I'm 68 years of age and, well, I've got problems with my private area.'

'Go on,' prompted the doctor.

'It's been painful passing water for several days,' explained Mr Donaldson. 'Now I've got this awful light green discharge coming from my privates. Oh and the pain when I pass water is unbearable. I hope you can get me better soon doctor, Mary and I always spend Tuesday afternoons together in her flat before going out for tea.'

'Let's begin by having a look at your private parts Mr Donaldson,' responded the doctor as he directed Mr Donaldson to the examination couch.

After examining Mr Donaldson the doctor asks: 'I know you're a single chap Mr Donaldson, but tell me, have you had any intimate relationships lately?'

Mr Donaldson laughs and replies, 'Well I did say the ladies are very agreeable and look after me, especially Mary. It's not special with the others like it is with Mary. Why do you ask doctor?'

'I think you may have gonorrhoea Mr Donaldson.'

Question one: Discuss sexually transmitted infections in relation to the elderly.

30 minutes

Question two: Explain what courses of action are open to the doctor and what health education and life-style changes the doctor might discuss with Mr Donaldson.

30 minutes

Time allowance: **1 hour**

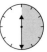

Answer to question one:
Discuss sexually transmitted infections in relation to the elderly.

A common misconception regarding elderly people is that they are sexually inactive when in fact as Mr Donaldson has demonstrated elderly people can still enjoy a satisfying love and sexual life (Brogan, 1996; Gibson, 1997; Grigg, 2000; Heath, 1999; Parke, 1991; Russell, 1998). As with any other age group who are sexually active, the elderly face the same risks of acquiring sexually transmitted infections (STIs), but health care professionals who do not regard the elderly as being sexually active may not imagine that they have acquired an STI (Grigg, 2000; Heath, 1999; Heath & Schofield, 1999; Heath, 2000).

It is difficult to estimate the number of elderly people who do acquire sexually transmitted infections. Figures for statistical analysis are collated from genito-urinary medicine clinics (who view older people as being over the age of 45) and few elderly people would be prepared to attend such clinics (Grigg, 2000). Most elderly patients, like Mr Donaldson, would prefer to visit their General Practitioner (Grigg, 2000).

Common health problems seen in the elderly such as arthritis, prostate or gynaecological problems may be the symptoms of untreated sexually transmitted infections, such as gonorrhoea (Grigg, 2000). Heath (2000, page 34) describes that the effect of untreated symptoms will be felt greater by the elderly because of the 'domino effect on their health'.

Marshall (1997) describes that 11% of people with Acquired Immune Deficiency Syndrome (AIDS) are over 50 years old and that this figure is increasing. Grigg (2000) estimates that there are around 10,000 elderly people in Britain who have undiagnosed Human Immunodeficiency Virus (HIV). This may be that symptoms such as weight loss, fatigue, weakness and anorexia often seen as signs of ageing could be HIV related illnesses (Heath, 1999; Heath & Schofield, 1999). AIDS related dementia can be misdiagnosed as Parkinson's disease or Alzheimer's disease (Tordoff, 1996; Whipple & Scura, 1996) and Grigg (2000) argues that Pneumocystis Carinii Pneumonia (PCP) could be misdiagnosed as Chronic Obstructive Airways Disease (COAD). Armstrong (2000) postulates that Syphilis induced confusion could be misdiagnosed as dementia.

Some authors argue that the elderly are at high risk of contracting sexually transmitted infections because they tend not to use contraceptive barrier methods (Grigg, 2000) such as condoms (Heath, 1999; Heath, 2000; Marshall, 1997) because there are no fears of unwanted pregnancy. However due to their reduced vaginal secretions and friable vaginal mucosa women are at greater risk of contracting an STI (Whipple & Scura, 1996).

Answer to question two:
Explain what courses of action are open to the doctor and what health education and life-style changes the doctor might discuss with Mr Donaldson.

Gonorrhoea is still the most common sexually transmitted infection (Grigg, 2000). The most effective treatment for gonorrhoea is antibiotics (Grigg, 2000; Kee & Hayes, 2000). Mr Donaldson's doctor may treat him at the surgery, or refer Mr Donaldson to a genito-urinary medicine clinic.

To reduce the risk of the spread of a sexually transmitted infection the doctor, or the staff at the genito-urinary medicine clinic will want to trace and treat all of Mr Donaldson's sexual contacts (Grigg, 2000; Kee & Hayes, 2000). Information exchanged will be treated confidentially, and contact names will not be revealed (Dimond, 1995).

The medical personnel treating Mr Donaldson and his sexual contacts will also screen for other sexually transmitted infections such as *Chlamydia trachomatis*, genital warts and syphilis (Grigg, 2000; Kee & Hayes, 2000). This should be followed by health advice regarding the risk of unprotected sex and the greater risk of STIs where multiple partners are involved, both of which may lead to sexually transmitted infections such as those screened for or others like HIV and AIDS (Kee & Hayes, 2000). The use of condoms treated with nonoxynol-9 to reduce the risk of an STI (Kee & Hayes, 2000) should be explained to Mr Donaldson and his sexual partners. This education may need to be extended into the correct use of a condom and how to apply and remove a condom safely.

Recent research has revealed that each act of coitus leaves tiny friction induced fissures on the surfaces of the vaginal wall and the glans of the penis which may aid the transmission of sexually acquired infections (Kee & Hayes, 2000). This problem will be exacerbated in the elderly person due to thinning of the vaginal wall and reduced vaginal lubrication (Eliopoulos, 1993; Grigg, 1999; Heath, 1999; Kee & Hayes, 2000; Parke, 1991; Russell, 1998). The medical personnel treating Mr Donaldson and his sexual partners could explain these natural changes to them.

Traditionally older people were not targeted for sexual health promotion campaigns. However new material is now being written specifically for the older person.

References

Armstrong, M. (2000) The pressures felt by informal carers of people with dementia. Nursing Standard 15(17): 47–53.
Brogan, M. (1996) The sexual needs of elderly people. Nursing Standard 10(24): 42–45.
Dimond, B. (1995) Legal Aspects of Nursing. (2nd ed.). London: Prentice Hall.
Eliopoulos, C. (1993) Gerontological Nursing. (3rd ed.). Philadelphia: J.B. Lippincott Company.
Gibson, H.B. (1997) Love in Later Life. London: Peter Owen.
Grigg, E. (1999) Sexuality and older people. Elderly Care 11(7): 12–15.
Grigg, E. (2000) Sexually transmitted infections and older people. Elderly Care 12(1): 15–19.

Heath, H. (1999) Sexuality in Old Age. NT Monographs No 40. London: Nursing Times Books.

Heath, H. (2000) Sexuality and continence in older women. Elderly Care 12(3): 32–34.

Heath, H., Schofield, I. (1999) (Ed.) Healthy Ageing: Nursing Older People. London: Mosby.

Kee, J.L., Hayes, E.R. (2000) Pharmacology: A Nursing Process Approach. (3rd ed.). London: W.B. Saunders Company.

Marshall, T. (1997) Infected and affected: HIV, AIDS and the older adult. Journal of the British Society of Gerontology 7(4): 8–11 cited by Grigg, E. (2000) Sexually transmitted infections and older people. Elderly Care 12(1): 15–19.

Parke, F. (1991) Sexuality in later life. Nursing Times 87(50): 40–42.

Russell, P. (1998) Sexuality in the lives of older people. Nursing Standard 13(8): 49–53.

Tordoff, C. (1996) The prevalence of HIV and AIDS in older people. Professional Nurse 12(3): 193–195 cited by Grigg, E. (2000) Sexually transmitted infections and older people. Elderly Care 12(1): 15–19.

Whipple, B., Scura, K. (1996) HIV in older adults. American Journal of Nursing 96(2): 23–28 cited by Heath, H. (2000) Sexuality and continence in older women. Elderly Care 12(3): 32–34.

Post-operative care following cardiac surgery

Lynn Randall

James Inglewood is a 65-year gentleman who lives with his wife Jean in a semi-detached house in a city. He has two children who are both married, live locally and visit infrequently.

James took early retirement 2 years ago due to restricted mobility resulting from increasing and persistent angina pectoris, accompanied with shortness of breath. He was employed as an electrician in the hosiery industry.

Prior to admission James' medication regime was daily aspirin 150 mg, 2 frumil tablets twice daily, 50 mg atenolol once daily, simvastatin 10 mg once daily, isosorbide mononitrite 60 mg once daily, and glyceryl trinitrite spray as necessary.

Three days ago James was admitted to a cardiac surgery unit for coronary artery bypass grafts (CABG). The day after admission he was transferred to theatre where he had a triple bypass graft consisting of two saphenous grafts, one to his right coronary artery (RCA), one to the obtuse marginal (OM) and the third graft was from the left internal mammary artery (LIMA) to the left anterior descending artery (LAD). His admission to the Cardiac Intensive Care unit was uneventful and he has subsequently been transferred back to the ward.

On admission to the ward James' baseline observations are: blood pressure (BP) 137/74 mmHg, heart rate 90 beats per minute. He has a temporary pacemaker in situ and he is receiving 2 litres of oxygen via nasal cannulae. He has one chest drain in the left pleural cavity, which is draining between 10 and 30 millilitres an hour.

Question one: Explain the specific post-operative complications that James is at risk of developing following cardiac surgery.

25 minutes

Question two: Postoperatively one of the specific complications can be pain. Can you identify the sites where this may occur and state possible interventions?

20 minutes

Question three: With reference to the case study list four areas which will need to be managed prior to discharge home.

20 minutes

Time allowance: **65 minutes**

Answer to question one:

Explain the specific post-operative complications that James is at risk of developing following cardiac surgery.

Cardiac surgical patients are generally cared for in either intensive care or high dependency environment during the first 12–24 hours post surgery thus providing one-to-one or one-to-two nurse to patient ratio. This provides an opportunity for close monitoring of the patient's physical condition and correction of any immediate complications of coronary artery bypass or non-bypass graft surgery (CABG/non-CABG).

There are a number of common complications with CABG surgery, these being in addition to the common post-operative surgical complications. These being:

- Rhythm disturbances
  - common arrhythmias include atrial fibrillation, atrioventricular (AV) blocks and ventricular ectopics
  - these are often as a result of hypothermia, altered potassium concentration and haemodilution
  - atrial arrhythmias occur in 11–40% of CABG, 2–3 days postoperatively (Ommen et al, 1997).
- Myocardial infarction
  - ST elevation can be due to occlusion or spasm of the grafted vessel
- Fluid management – dehydration/fluid overload
  - blood loss can occur intra-operatively
  - fluid replacement is dependant on a number of factors:
    - low BP, increased heart rate, decreased central venous pressure (CVP) and haemoglobin (Hb)/haematocrit
  - the choice of fluid will be reflected in these parameters and the patient's general condition
  - blood will increase the oxygen delivery and exert oncotic pressure thereby reducing interstitial oedema in comparison to colloids (Kavanagh et al, 1995); however there are infection risks with its use.
- Cardiac tamponade
  - The accumulation of blood or serous fluid around the heart, usually in the pericardial sac. The fluid constricts the pumping action of the heart and leads to haemodynamic collapse.
  - The patient initially presents with a rise in CVP as pressure constricts the heart. The BP falls, heart rate increasing tachycardia and if there are chest drains in situ the drainage will slow or stop.
  - In surgical emergency the patient will be returned to theatre, re-opened to evacuate the blood and repair the cause of the bleed.
- Post-operative pain
  - pain can vary between patients, it is however important to distinguish between incisional pain and ischaemic pain
- Barotrauma – pneumothorax
  - during the period of cardiopulmonary bypass surgery the lungs are deflated and the flow of blood bypasses them

- – the chest drains inserted at the end of the operation allow the blood which collects in the pericardial space after the operation to drain freely
  - – pneumothorax/haemothorax can occur
- Renal effects
  - – at the commencement of cardiopulmonary bypass (CPB) there is a decrease in renal blood flow
  - – large quantities of fluid are required to maintain the CPB circuit
  - – these factors increase the incidence of acute renal failure especially with patients with pre-existing renal failure
- Raised blood glucose and unstable diabetes
  - – can be as a result of the use of inotropic therapy
- Confessional states/post-pump delirium
  - – altered neurological function is common in general surgical procedures
  - – with CPB also associated with memory loss and mild personality changes (Tucker, 1993).
- Cerebrovascular accident
  - – the result of the combination of anaesthesia, surgical insult, coagulation abnormalities and CPB
- Late post-operative anaemia – blood transfusion
  - – low Hb and haematocrit at discharge, needs checking and treating prior to discharge

(Adapted from Fisher et al, 2002)

Answer to question two:
Postoperatively one of the specific complications can be pain. Can you identify the sites where this may occur and state possible interventions?

Post-operative pain will vary between patients. However, with pain following cardiac surgery it is important to distinguish between incisional and ischaemic pain. The pain experienced following cardiac surgery relates to:

* the location and type of surgery
* intra-operative manipulation of the heart and lungs
* presence of invasive lines and chest drains.

  The possible sites of pain are:

* the median stenotomy
    – pain may be experienced along the stenotomy wound – this can generally be differentiated from post-operative recurrent angina pain because it is not related to exercise, it is exacerbated by changes in position and there is often associated numbness to the skin of the chest wall.
* leg saphenous vein graft site.

De Laria et al (1981) indicate that harvesting the entire saphenous vein can leave the longest operative incision used for an operation. Once mobilisation has commenced it is a common site for pain, which is often accompanied with oedema and numbness along the harvest site.

Other complications associated with this site include delayed healing. This can be related to a number of risk factors such as diabetes mellitus, peripheral vascular disease, smoking, obesity and may also relate to poor harvesting techniques:

* Graft sites of the radial arteries
* Sites of lines and drains
    – urinary catheter, central/peripheral lines, chest drains and vacuum drains.

The management of the pain will depend on the type of the pain and the site of the pain experienced. Hancock (1996) suggests that adequate pain relief depends on the individual's perception of pain rather than on the precise nature of the surgery. The analgesic regimen for non-ischaemic pain is normally a combination of:
    – opioids – morphine
    – non-opioids – paracetamol, dihydrocodeine
    – non-steroidal anti inflammatory drugs – diclofenac (these are used with caution as they can affect the renal function).

(Adapted from Hancock, 1996)

Answer to question three:
With reference to the case study list four areas which will need to be managed prior to discharge home.

The following areas will need to be managed prior to discharge home:

- Removal of chest drains
  - The chest drains are normally removed after the first 24 hours post surgery or when the drainage is less than 100 ml in the previous 4–6 hours according to the surgeon's preference. The drains cause the patient discomfort when in situ and restrict adequate chest expansion.
  - Patients require adequate analgesia if chest drains are in situ and during removal of the drains.
  - The drains should be removed following local policy.
- Removal of central lines
  - generally the central lines are left in place until the 2nd post-operative day
  - ensuring the patient is cardiovascularly stable prior to their removal
  - the central line should be removed following local policy.
- Removal of pacing wires
  - If the heart rate is judged to be adequate to maintain blood pressure, the pacing box will be turned off for a period of 24–48 hours at which time the medical staff will instruct the pacing wires to be removed.
  - The clotting status will be confirmed prior to removal of the wires. If the clotting is abnormal the medical staff will prescribe the relevant clotting products to be given prior to removal.
  - A complication of their removal is bleeding around the heart.
  - The pacing wires should be removed following local policy.
- Education to James and his wife into the regimen of drugs he will go home with. James' medications may well have changed; it is important that he understands the medication he will be taking, their actions, the doses and when they need to be taken. The possible side effects should also be discussed with them.

References

De Laria, G.A., Hunter, J.A., Goldin, M.D., Serry, C., Javid, H., Najafi, H. (1981) Leg wound complications associated with coronary revascularisation. Journal of Thoracic and Cardiovascular Surgery 81(3): 403–407.

Fisher, S., Walsh, G., Cross, N. (2002) Chapter 22 'Nursing management of the cardiac surgical patient' in Hatchett, R., Thompson, D. Cardiac Nursing – A Comprehensive Guide. Edinburgh: Churchill Livingstone.

Hancock, H. (1996) The complexity of pain assessment and management in the first 24 hours after cardiac surgery: implications for nurses. Part 1. Intensive and Critical Care Nursing 12: 295–302.

Kavanagh, R., Radhakrishnan, D., Park, G. (1995) Crystalloids and colloids in the critically ill patient. Care of the Critically Ill 11(3): 114–119.

Milner, R., Treasure, T. (1995) Explaining Cardiac Surgery – Patient Assessment and Care. BMJ Publishing Group.

Ommen, S., Odell, J., Stanton, M. (1997) Atrial arrhythmias after cardiothoracic surgery. New England Journal of Medicine 336(20): 1429–1434.

Tucker, L.A. (1993) Post-pump delirium. Intensive and Critical Care Nursing 9(4): 269–273.

Further reading

Department of Health (2000) National Service Framework – Coronary Heart Disease – Modern Standards and Service Models. Department of Health Publication.

Hatchett, R., Thompson, D. (2002) Cardiac Nursing – A Comprehensive Guide. Edinburgh: Churchill Livingstone.

Laparoscopic cholecystectomy

Liz Shears & Julia Ball

Rachel White is 34 years old and the mother of two young children aged 6 years and 18 months. Her husband is a police officer who works shifts, however she manages to work 20 hours a week in the local supermarket as she receives help with child care from her mother and two sisters who live nearby.

Over the last 3 months, Rachel has noticed an increasing intolerance to fatty foods in her diet with a vague discomfort in her right hypochondrium. Recently this discomfort has increased in intensity with pain radiating up to her back and right shoulder with accompanying nausea and vomiting. After consulting her General Practitioner (GP) she was referred to the local hospital for an ultrasound scan, the result of which confirmed the presence of gallstones in her gallbladder.

Rachel is to be admitted to your ward for a laparoscopic cholecystectomy intended as a day case and is prepared accordingly. Having always been relatively healthy, with no previous illnesses, this is her first time in hospital, except for when she was having her children. When she returns to the ward from the operating theatre she has a small vacuum drain in situ and it is necessary for her to stay in hospital overnight, with discharge home anticipated for the following morning.

Question one: What criteria would make Rachel suitable for day case surgery?

15 minutes

Question two: What are the nursing priorities in caring for Rachel on her return to the ward from the operating theatre until her discharge?

25 minutes

Question three: What information should Rachel receive prior to discharge home?

20 minutes

Time allowance: **60 minutes**

Answer to question one:
What criteria would make Rachel suitable for day case surgery?

There are criteria for selecting patients for day case surgery and with developments in techniques and anaesthesia there is increasing flexibility that more patients can access this type of surgery (Malster & Parry, 2000). Such assessment can include:

Psychological assessment

- Rachel must want to be treated as a day case and understand the implications of being treated as such.
- She may be asked to sign a patient agreement acknowledging the terms agreed for day surgery such as not to drink alcohol, drive, cycle or operate machinery for at least 24 hours postoperatively.

Social assessment

- Rachel must be collected from the ward or unit by a responsible adult who will provide transport (public transport is not recommended).
- A responsible adult must remain with Rachel for at least 24 hours after her operation. She will need to have made arrangements for childcare.
- Easy access to a toilet is required and a telephone.

Physical assessment

- Rachel will have her weight recorded for the purpose of calculating drugs that she may receive. A body mass index (BMI) will indicate if the patient is obese and the potential threat to their health.
- Blood pressure and pulse rate will also be taken at the pre-assessment clinic to identify actual disorders such as hypertension and to utilise as a baseline so that changes can be quickly identified postoperatively.
- Any medication will be noted. The oral contraceptive pill may be stopped after discussion with the surgeon as there is a risk of abnormal blood clotting. Advice should be given to Rachel regarding alternative contraception.
- Normally only patients who are classified ASA I (normal healthy adult) or ASA II (a patient with a mild systemic disease) are considered suitable for day case anaesthesia. The ASA III category are patients with a severe systemic disease which limits activity.
- Allergies must be recorded and those with a latex allergy are not suitable to be treated as a day case.

(Adapted from Royal College of Surgeons, 1992)

Answer to question two:
What are the nursing priorities in caring for Rachel on her return to the ward from the operating theatre until her discharge?

- Observations of temperature, pulse and blood pressure as clinically indicated to detect any complications, such as haemorrhage or infection.
- Observing conscious level and respiratory rate, to monitor the recovery of the patient from the anaesthetic gases. Once Rachel is awake she can be nursed in an upright position to facilitate deep breathing exercises and lung expansion.
- Pain relief should be administered as prescribed and Rachel should be monitored for the effectiveness of the medication. This will help to maintain Rachel's comfort and facilitate deep breathing exercises and early mobilisation. Rachel may experience shoulder tip pain from the residual carbon dioxide, used during the operation to dilate her abdomen, collecting under her diaphragm and irritating the phrenic nerve (Parboteeah, 1998).
- Observe the four puncture sites for any excessive bleeding onto the dressings.
- Ensure that the vacuum drain is functional (that there is a vacuum present and that the tubes are unclamped), noting the amount and type of drainage to detect for excessive bleeding or the presence of bile.
- The drain should be removed prior to Rachel's discharge after having first explained the procedure to her, ensured that the vacuum is released on the drainage bottle (according to manufacturer's instructions) and that an analgesic has been given if required. A dressing should be applied to the site.
- Rachel may have an intravenous infusion in situ on return to the ward. This can be discontinued as soon as she can tolerate fluids, which should be within a few hours of returning to the ward. She can also take diet as tolerated after this time.
- If Rachel is nauseated or vomiting, administer anti-emetics as prescribed, and monitor effect.
- To reduce the risk of deep vein thrombosis Rachel should have anti-embolism stockings, low molecular heparin injections and be encouraged to mobilise at the earliest opportunity.
- Urinary output should be monitored postoperatively and Rachel should pass urine within 8 hours (Williamson, 1998).

Answer to question three:
What information should Rachel receive prior to discharge home?

- Provision of appropriate analgesic for the following few days and giving advice if this analgesic is likely to cause side effects. A letter should be provided for her GP outlining her hospital treatment.
- Advice on wound care. The small dressings can be removed on the third day noting any redness or leaking from sites. Arrangements should be made for Rachel to visit the practice nurse for her clips or sutures to be removed 7–10 days postoperatively.
- Rachel should be advised to consult her GP if she experiences an increase in pain, develops a rise in temperature, calf pain or a productive cough. (The potential complications following surgery may be a bile leak, wound or chest infection or deep vein thrombosis.)
- Rachel should be able to resume normal activities over the next 5–7 days, whilst care should be taken to avoid lifting heavy weights at home or at work for the next few weeks to minimise complications. Rachel may need providing with a sickness certificate to cover her absence from work.
- Transport arrangements for Rachel should be confirmed.
- Rachel is advised that driving may be possible after a couple of weeks, or whenever she can control the car comfortably and safely (including emergency stop). This time will vary depending on the individual and their recovery from the surgery.

References

Malster, M., Parry, A. (2000) Ch. 15. Day surgery. In: Manley, K., Bellman, L. (Eds) Surgical Nursing Advancing Practice. Edinburgh: Churchill Livingstone.

Parboteeah, S. (1998) Ch. 8. Gastrointestinal surgery. In: Simpson, P.M. (Ed.) Introduction to Surgical Nursing. London: Arnold.

Royal College of Surgeons (1992) Report of the Working Party Guidelines for Day Case Surgery. London: HMSO.

Williamson, L. (1998) Post-operative care, Part II (Practical procedures for nurses, Part 11.2). Nursing Times 94(12).

Further reading

Cassidy, J., Marley, R. (1996) Preoperative assessment of the ambulatory patient. Journal of Peri-Anaesthesia Nursing 11(5): 334–343.

Department of Health (2000) The NHS Plan. London: HMSO Or www.nhs.uk/nationalplan

Dutton, K., Waters, G. (2000) Ch. 7. Day surgery. In: Pudner R. (Ed.) Nursing the surgical patient. Edinburgh: Bailliere Tindall/RCN.

Mallett, J., Dougherty, L. (2000) The Royal Marsden Hospital Manual of Clinical Nursing Procedures. (5th ed.). Oxford: Blackwell Science.

Mitchell, M. (2002) Guidance for the psychological care of day case surgery patients. Nursing Standard 16(40): 41–43.

Upper gastrointestinal tract bleed (peptic ulcer)

Penny Harrison

Mr Maurice Kavanagh, is a 68-year-old widower, who lives alone in his bungalow with his two cats. His daughters live in another city and visit for long weekends. Maurice is relatively independent with his activities of living, including washing, dressing, shopping, cooking, cleaning and gardening. Maurice relies on his daughters and their families to do the heavier gardening such as weeding/sweeping and housework such as cleaning the windows. Maurice goes out twice a week to the local club where he meets with friends and acquaintances. Maurice is of slightly above average weight for his height and enjoys a good diet as well as four pints of beer when he goes to the club. Maurice has previously smoked, but now only consumes a cigar on special occasions.

Maurice's previous medical history includes suffering from a small myocardial infarction and a stroke, from which he has made a full recovery. Amongst a range of medications taken to manage his cardiovascular function, Maurice takes aspirin 150 mg daily. Maurice also suffers with arthritis, with some stiffness and pain in his shoulders and hips. Despite this Maurice has been very determined to live a full and active life. For the last 12 months his arthritis has warranted taking regular analgesic drugs to reduce the pain, inflammation and stiffness in his joints. This has generally been very effective, although Maurice sometimes forgets to take his medication as prescribed and catches up with his breakfast dose later in the morning.

Recently Maurice has been to see his General Practitioner (GP) complaining of a range of symptoms including indigestion, heartburn, acid reflux and acute abdominal pain. These symptoms sometimes resolve independently or are reduced by drinking a milky coffee. Maurice's GP referred him to the local hospital where an oesophagogastroduodenoscopy (OGD) was performed. This revealed a large gastric ulcer with evidence of recent bleeding. Maurice has completed the initial course of treatment for the *Helicobacter pylori* bacteria (*H. pylori*), as biopsies at the time of the original OGD showed that this bacteria was present in Maurice's stomach. Maurice is continuing with treatment to assist his gastric ulcer to heal. Maurice is due for a repeat OGD within the next 12 weeks to check that the gastric ulcer has healed. However, Maurice has had to be admitted to the emergency medical ward, as he has had a large gastric bleed. Maurice vomited up copious amounts of blood, with loss estimated to be about 1500 millilitres, and was in a shocked state with a blood pressure of 80/60 mmHg and a pulse of 140 beats per minute.

Question one: What is a peptic ulcer and what risk factors does Maurice have that would pre dispose him to developing such an ulcer?

20 minutes

Question two: What treatments are available to minimise further bleeding and to promote healing of Maurice's gastric ulcer?

20 minutes

Question three: What are the key aspects of nursing care for Maurice on admission?

30 minutes

Time allowance: **70 minutes**

Answer to question one:
What is a peptic ulcer and what risk factors does Maurice have that would pre dispose him to developing such an ulcer?

Peptic disease is a broad term that refers to any area of the gastrointestinal tract that has been damaged by acid and pepsin-containing secretions. Thus the terms gastric erosions, gastric ulceration and duodenal ulceration are included by this term (Elliot, 2002). Peptic ulcers give individuals unpleasant symptoms. They also have the potential to cause life threatening emergencies frequently by causing erosion of the mucosal epithelium and blood vessels.

The stomach and duodenum are key parts of the gastrointestinal tract that are responsible for specific functions for digestion of food ingested. The fundus of the stomach (Fig. 25.1) acts as a reservoir for storage of food as it enters the stomach. The body of the stomach mixes food with gastric secretions to form chyme. The antrum of the stomach propels the chyme via the pylorus towards the duodenum. The four layers of the stomach are designed for mixing and digestion of food. The stomach has a high pH of two, with an acidic environment. The cells of the wall of the stomach are made up largely from proteins to assist with protection from auto digestion. Factors that breach this protection cause ulceration of the stomach mucosa (Elliot, 2002).

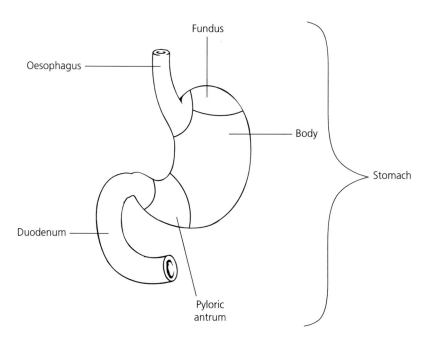

Figure 25.1: Sections of the stomach.

There are three common causes of upper gastrointestinal bleeding:

H. pylori

H. pylori is a bacteria discovered in the 1980s (Tsai, 1997) and is believed to be a key factor in the development of gastric and duodenal ulceration. The bacteria lodges itself in the mucous of the stomach. The stomach is usually too acidic for bacteria, but H. pylori has a number of features that has enabled it to adjust to the acidic environment of this part of the gastrointestinal tract (Elliot, 2002). Thus H. pylori causes chronic infection, with symptoms of inflammation or gastritis. H. pylori are believed to be acquired in childhood via the oral–oral or faecal–oral route.

Non-steroidal anti inflammatory drugs (NSAIDs)

NSAIDs are thought to be factors that contribute to the development of ulcers. This is due to the damage that is caused to the mucosa of the stomach by reduction in the production of prostaglandin secretion. These protect the mucosa of the stomach from auto digestion by the gastric secretions. NSAID and aspirin are widely prescribed for a wide range of patients and conditions, especially older patients (Butler, 1997). Maurice takes NSAIDs for pain management for his arthritis and aspirin for its anti clotting effect on platelets to protect his cardiovascular system from further episodes such as stroke and myocardial infarction. Patients are advised to take these medicines with or soon after food to assist with protection of the mucosa of the stomach. Maurice sometimes forgets to take his morning medication with breakfast. The nurse is well placed to advise on strategies to assist with this, reinforcing the importance of taking NSAIDs with food.

Stress

Life events that create stress are thought to be a contributory cause towards ulceration of the upper gastrointestinal tract. However this remains controversial as difficulties remain in defining stress and relating this to ulcer disease (Butler, 1997). Maurice may have stress in his life from continuing to try to remain independent as possible. The nurse is well placed to co-ordinate a full multi-professional assessment of the patient's abilities and likely future needs prior to discharge, ensuring that Maurice's wishes are central to any decisions taken.

Other risk factors

Smoking increases acid production which in turn increases the risk of epithelial damage (Butler, 1997). Maurice previously smoked and occasionally smokes currently. The nurse can advise on the risks of continuing to smoke intermittently.

Alcohol and other contents of the diet such as excessive coffee may act as a direct irritant to the lining of the stomach, causing erosion which may lead to ulceration (Butler, 1997). Maurice ingests beer in some quantity twice weekly. Maurice cooks his own food, which may be high in food types such as fat or sugar that require a large amount of gastric secretions to commence the process of digestion, hence increasing the risk of gastric erosion. The nurse is well placed to complete a nutritional and lifestyle assessment relating to diet and alcohol. Referral to the dietician may be helpful for further specialist advice.

Answer to question two:
What treatments are available to minimise further bleeding and to promote healing of Maurice's gastric ulcer?

The aim of therapeutic interventions are to reduce the risk of further bleeding and this may be achieved by medical intervention which includes injection – epinephrine (adrenaline) solution or other agents are used to cause the ulcer or bleeding point to sclerose. Thus the ulcer will gradually be reduced in size, and will be less likely to bleed.

- Laser treatment – the laser is used for photo-coagulation. Any bleeding points will be coagulated, reducing the risk of bleeding.
- Injection therapy – this will cause vasoconstriction and thrombosis with secondary surrounding fibrosis.

These treatments are administered via an endoscope. (Nursing details of caring for a patient requiring an endoscopy is in Case 11).

- Surgical intervention – if unresponsive to the above treatment surgical intervention might be considered to maintain haemostasis.
- Drug therapy – this may comprise a combination of drugs. This may include two types of antibiotic (one broad spectrum for example Clarithromycin, an anaerobic antibiotic such as Metronidazole). In addition an ulcer healing drug such as Lansoprazole) completes the drug regimen.

As Maurice has evidence of a gastric ulcer from his first OGD, he will be prescribed drug therapy to eradicate the *H. pylori* bacteria and then continue on his ulcer healing drug until his subsequent OGD, when the gastric ulcer can be reassessed for its progress in healing.

Answers to question three:
What are the key aspects of nursing care for Maurice on admission?

Patients who present with an acute upper gastrointestinal bleed are in a life threatening condition, requiring urgent assessment and resuscitation to correct the effects of hypovolaemic shock. For Maurice, this requires the following nursing interventions:

Observations

Recording of blood pressure, pulse, respiration, oxygen saturation and noting the level of pallor will be performed on admission and then as clinically indicated. This is a key tool in assessing for hypovolaemic shock (Case 3).

Fluid management

The monitoring and replacement of fluids is a fundamental aspect in managing Maurice's care. The nurse will need to record episodes of vomiting, colour and consistency of the vomit, estimated loss of blood in haematemesis, record all input of intravenous fluids administered including whole blood and blood products such as plasma, as well as additional fluids such as synthetic plasma expanders.

A central venous catheter may be inserted to enable fluids to be administered rapidly and to monitor central venous pressure. The nurse is well placed to oversee that local policies are followed, even in the emergency medical ward, to ensure safe transfusion of blood. (For more details on the role of the nurse in blood transfusion, refer to Case 20). The nurse can also assist Maurice with oral hygiene following episodes of haematemesis, ensuring that vomit bowl, tissues and call bell are close at hand.

Urinary catheterisation may be necessary if the patient is showing signs of developing hypovolaemic shock.

Oral intake restriction

It is imperative that Maurice takes no fluids or any other substance by mouth whilst he is actively bleeding and until his condition has been stabilised. This is to allow for an OGD to assess the nature of Maurice's bleeding and the likelihood of gastric surgery and general anaesthesia.

Communication/reassurance to patient and family

Maurice will be frightened by the vomiting and loss of blood. He and his family will require the nurse to communicate information about what is happening and the likely interventions to stabilise the bleeding. The nurse is also able to liaise between the multi disciplinary team to ensure safe transfer between the ward and endoscopy unit, if OGD is to be undertaken, or the ward and operating theatres in anticipation of preparation for surgery.

References

Butler, M. (1997) (Eds) Gastrointestinal bleeding. In Bruce, L., Finlay, T. Nursing in Gastroenterology. Edinburgh: Churchill Livingstone.
Cotrill, M. (1996) *Helicobacter pylori*. Professional Nurse 12(1): 46–48.
Cotton, P., Williams, C. (1996) Practical Gastrointestinal Endoscopy. (4th ed.). Oxford: Blackwell Scientific.
D'Silva, J. (1998) Upper gastrointestinal endoscopy: gastroscopy. Nursing Standard 12(45): 49–56.
Elliot, D. (2002) The treatment of peptic ulcers. Nursing Standard 16(22): 37–42.
Tsai, H. (1997) *H. pylori* for the general physician. Journal of the Royal College of Physicians of London 31(5): 478–482.

Further reading

Alexander, M., Fawcett, J., Runciman, P. (2000) Nursing Practice Hospital and Home: The Adult. Edinburgh: Churchill Livingstone.
Hicks, S. (2000) Gastric cancer: diagnosis, risk factors, treatment and life issues. British Journal of Nursing 10(8): 529–536.
National Institute for Clinical Excellence (2000) Guidance on the use of proton pump inhibitors. London: NICE.

Exhibitionism/masturbation Alzheimer's Disease

Chris Buswell

'Do you mind if we both go and assist Mr Pringle to the toilet Cath, only he gives me the creeps sometimes?'

'Sure Sarah, I think I know just how you feel. I remember when I first met him, he was sat next to Mrs Booth with his arms around her. Well I naturally assumed it was his wife come to visit him and they were just being affectionate to each other. Imagine when the next minute Mrs Pringle did arrive. I tell you that was an embarrassing moment. Mrs Pringle didn't seem to understand when the nurse said that Mr Pringle could have mistaken Mrs Booth for his wife because of his Alzheimer's Disease.'

'Gosh Cath, you'd think at 82 years old one woman would be enough' laughed Sarah.

'Yes, but he's getting worse I think. Ever since the doctor last saw him. I mean I'm no nurse but I'm sure those new tablets of his have affected him in an area old men shouldn't be affected.'

'You're right there Cath, why only last week his hands started wondering while I was washing him down below. It really upset me. When I mentioned it to the nurse in charge of the shift she just laughed.'

As carers Cath and Sarah walk into the lounge of the nursing home they are aghast to find Mr Pringle openly masturbating in the presence of three frightened women patients. They scold Mr Pringle for his behaviour and take him to his room, where he spends the rest of the day in solitude.

Question one: Discuss exhibitionism/masturbation in relation to the male patient with Alzheimer's Disease.

Time allowance: **50 minutes**

Answer to question one:
Discuss exhibitionism/masturbation in relation to the male patient with Alzheimer's Disease.

A significant part of healthy ageing is the appropriate expression of sexuality (Brogan, 1996; Drench & Losee, 1996; Eliopoulos, 1993; Gibson, 1997a; Heath, 1999; Heath & Schofield, 1999; Heath & White, 2001).

In the scenario described above the most important point to remember is that Mr Pringle suffers from Alzheimer's Disease. Due to this he may not be able to identify correct and appropriate expression of sexuality (Armstrong, 2000; Kuhn, Greiner & Arseneau, 1998). He may indeed have mistaken Mrs Booth for his wife. It is common for patients in care homes to mistake other patients as their spouses or lovers due to impaired memory, judgement and insight (Kuhn, Greiner & Arseneau, 1998). Staff in nursing and residential homes must remain alert to this problem for the safety and dignity of all their patients.

When the carer was washing Mr Pringle's genitalia he may have imagined a sexual encounter, due to his lack of understanding and insight. When Mr Pringle was masturbating inappropriately in the lounge he may have thought he was alone.

Commonly in Alzheimer's Disease some patients may lose their sexual inhibitions and display inappropriate behaviour (Armstrong, 2000; Smith, 2000; Wilcock, 1999). It is thought to be due to damage to the frontal and temporal lobes of the brain which regulate libido, such as in Pick's Disease (Kuhn, Greiner & Arseneau, 1998; Smith, 2000; Wilcock, 1999). Other patients with Alzheimer's Disease may lose all interest in sexual activity (Smith, 2000).

However all patients with Alzheimer's Disease, and their spouses/partners, still have sexual needs and feelings (Wilcock, 1999). Individualised care and care planning regarding sexuality should be openly discussed between the patient and his or her loved one and the care team. Spouses or partners of a patient with Alzheimer's Disease should be encouraged to maintain normal loving and physical relationships. Staff can facilitate this by providing privacy times and acting non judgementally without exhibiting their own prejudices. Matrons and managers of care homes are in an ideal position to influence their staff by running training sessions regarding sexuality of the elderly. Such training programmes could involve exercises in self reflection to help staff overcome their fears and prejudices concerning love and sexuality in later life. Such training could extend to all staff in care homes who may have contact with patients and their loved ones, such as cleaners and administrators, so that a multi disciplinary understanding and approach can be implemented.

Some patients with Alzheimer's may choose to masturbate, albeit in public rather than in private. Eliopoulos (1993) and Gibson (1997b) consider masturbation to be beneficial in releasing sexual tensions whilst maintaining the continued function of the genitalia. Kellett (1993) considers masturbation to be a healthy practice in later life, especially for people who have no sexual partner. Nurses have a duty to patients who wish to masturbate to provide privacy and dignity whilst maintaining non judgemental attitudes which prevent feelings of guilt or abnormality by the patient (Aylott, 1998; Eliopoulos, 1993; Gibson, 1997b).

Shelton (1992) describes a patient who would inappropriately masturbate by lying on a cold hard floor and rock from side to side in an effort to ejaculate. During this action the friction would result in the patient suffering burns and open wounds to his stomach and thighs and bleeding to his penis. The multi disciplinary team caring for the patient assessed the patient and implemented a plan which involved verbal and physical techniques of teaching the patient to masturbate more appropriately in the privacy of his own room. This resulted in the patient spending less time masturbating and a reduction in self injury. Aylott (1998) argues that it is a nursing duty to teach patients to express their sexuality appropriately and that nurses may professionally overlap their role with that of a sex therapist. The nursing staff and the matron of the nursing home in which Mr Pringle lived may have felt it appropriate and felt competent enough to allow Mr Pringle to masturbate in the privacy of his bedroom and within the constraints of his Alzheimer's Disease if Mr Pringle has enough insight, to teach him not to masturbate in the lounge. The nursing staff should also arrange for a medication review since some drugs, such as Levodopa, can cause hypersexuality (Weinman & Ruskin, 1995). Kuhn, Greiner and Arseneau (1998) advocate a full medical examination by the patient's doctor since not all inappropriate sexual behaviour is due to dementia, but can be attributed to another physical cause. Not all inappropriate action of a patient with Alzheimer's Disease can be sexual in origin. For example Wilcock (1999) describes a gentleman who removed his trousers in public because he was trying to communicate that he needed to void urine but had forgotten how to get to the toilet and that he should undress in the toilet and not in the prescence of others. One solution that Wilcock (1999) offers is to dress patients who exhibit such behaviour in trousers with velcro fastenings at the back. Other authors also advocate modifying clothing so that the patient finds it difficult to remove it (Kuhn, Greiner & Arseneau, 1998).

The Alzheimer patient may be seeking love, comfort and closeness, but inappropriately displays this as sexual aggression due to a lack of self awareness and inhibitions that would normally restrain sexual urges (Kuhn, Greiner & Arseneau, 1998). Other Alzheimer sufferers may just seek physical contact such as hand holding but display this as fondling other parts of their and other people's bodies (Kuhn, Greiner & Arseneau, 1998).

Some patients with Alzheimer's Disease may be simply bored and are exploring their bodies as a form of self stimulation (Kuhn, Greiner & Arseneau, 1998). Staff in nursing and residential homes can play an active part in diverting patients' attentions to fulfilling hobbies and interests or group activity times. Some homes employ a specific person, often called an activity co-ordinator, to assist patients with leisurely pursuits. Mr Pringle may not respond well to being isolated in his room by the staff and might benefit from structured and organised activity time either in a one to one situation or in a group.

References

Armstrong, M. (2000) The pressures felt by informal carers of people with dementia. Nursing Standard 15(17): 47–53.

Aylott, J. (1998) Sense and sexuality. Nursing Times 94(23): 34–35.

Brogan, M. (1996) The sexual needs of elderly people. Nursing Standard 10(24): 42–45.

Drench, M.E., Losee, R.H. (1996) Sexuality and sexual capacities in elderly people. Rehabilitation Nursing 21(3): 118–123.

Eliopoulos, C. (1993) Gerontological Nursing. (3rd ed.). Philadelphia: J.B. Lippincott Company.

Gibson, H.B. (1997a) Love in later life. London: Peter Owen.

Gibson, H.B. (1997b) A Little of What You Fancy Does You Good: Your Health in Later Life. London: Third Age Press.

Heath, H. (1999) Sexuality in Old Age. NT Monograph No 40. London: NT Books.

Heath, H., Schofield, I. (1999) (Ed) Healthy Ageing: Nursing Older People. London: Mosby.

Heath, H., White, I. (2001) Sexuality and older people: an introduction to nursing. Nursing Older People 13(4): 29–31.

Kellett, J. (1993) Sexuality in later life. Rev Clin Gerontol 3: 309–314 cited by Heath, H., Schofield, I. (1999) Healthy Ageing: Nursing Older People. London: Mosby.

Kuhn, D.R., Greiner, D., Arseneau, L. (1998) Addressing Hypersexuality in Alzheimer's Disease. Journal of Gerontological Nursing 24(4): 44–50.

Shelton, D. (1992) Client sexual behaviour and staff attitudes: shaping masturbation in an individual with a profound mental and secondary sensory handicap. Mental Handicap 20(2): 81–84 cited in Aylott, J. (1998). Sense and sexuality. Nursing Times 94(23): 34–35.

Smith, T. (2000) Living with Alzheimer's Disease. London: Sheldon Press.

Weinman, E., Ruskin, P.E. (1995) Levodopa dependence and hypersexuality in an older Parkinson's disease patient. American Journal of Geriatric Psychiatry 3(1): 81–83 cited by Kuhn, D.R., Greiner, D., Arseneau, L. (1998) Addressing Hypersexuality in Alzheimer's Disease. Journal of Gerontological Nursing 24(4): 44–50.

Wilcock, G. (1999) Living with Alzheimer's Disease and Similar Conditions. London: Penguin Books Ltd.

Myocardial infarction

Penny Tremayne

Ranjit Patel is a 48-year-old shop owner married to Amerjit. They have four children aged 21, 19, 17 and 13 years all who live at home together with Amerjit's 76-year-old widowed mother. Ranjit and his family live in a large detached house which is only a 5 minute drive from the shop.

Ranjit arrives at his shop at 5.00 a.m. every day to receive deliveries of newspapers. He works behind the shop counter and is responsible for the day to day running of this popular and successful business. His family are very supportive, each member assisting in the shop at some point during the day. Although he employs two part-time staff, Ranjit often does not get home until after 8.00 p.m. Recently he has become worried about the prospect of a competitive hypermarket opening nearby.

He has no time for hobbies as such, but enjoys spending time with his family and watching television.

One morning Ranjit experiences indigestion type pain. He drinks a glass of milk and thinks nothing more of it. That afternoon however, while stacking shelves Ranjit experiences a crushing band of burning pain in his chest that radiates down his left shoulder and arm, neck and lower jaw. He shouts for attention before lowering himself to the floor. Fortunately, a member of staff quickly attends to Ranjit and phones for an ambulance.

Meanwhile, Ranjit who is sweating profusely complains of nausea and promptly vomits. The pain is excrutiating, he feels as though there is an unbearable pressure across his chest and he cries 'this is the end'.

On arrival the paramedics take Ranjit's history, record an electrocardio-gram (ECG) which shows changes; they also take recordings of temperature (T) which is 38.5°C, pulse (P) rate is 117 beats per minute, respiratory (R) rate is 24 per minute, Blood Pressure (BP) is 90/50 mmHg and oxygen satur-ation is 87%. These all contribute to a provisional diagnosis of an acute myocardial infarction. A high concentration of oxygen is given, diamorphine 5 mg is given for pain relief alongside metoclopramide 10 mg, an anti emetic and aspirin 300 mg is administered orally.

As his condition is briefly stabilised, Ranjit is transferred to the Hospital's Coronary Care Unit.

Question one: Explain what a myocardial infarction is.

15 minutes

Question two: What initial investigations will be undertaken?

10 minutes

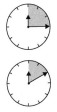

Question three: Explain the initial medical and nursing interventions on arrival to hospital.

20 minutes

Question four: Outline the role of thrombolysis and list the contraindicators and complications of its use.

15 minutes

Time allowance: **60 minutes**

Answer to question one:
Explain what a myocardial infarction is.

A myocardial infarction involves the destruction of myocardial tissue as a result of a blockage in the supply of blood and therefore oxygen via the coronary arteries. It can occur as a consequence of the following:

- Atherosclerosis – '…the accumulation of lipid deposits in the intima of the coronary arteries (Fig. 27.1), eventually forming atheromatous plaques that obstruct the flow of blood' (Pearson, 1999, 44).
- Thrombosis – the more likely cause of a myocardial infarction is when the atherosclerotic plaque ruptures inappropriate clotting and subsequent occlusion of the coronary artery (Hand, 2001).
- Severe coronary artery spasm – Hand (2001) indicates that this little understood condition can even affect atherosclerotic and non-atherosclerotic coronary arteries. Spasm reduces the blood flow through the coronary arteries and therefore there is an increased risk of thrombosis.

Regions of the heart that can be affected by an infarction include:

- Anterior – the front of the heart
- Lateral – left side of the heart
- Anterolateral – front and side of the heart
- Septal – central area of the heart
- Inferior – lower area of the heart
- Posterior – back of the heart
- Posterolateral – side through to the back of the heart

Hatchett (2001)

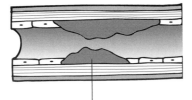

Atherosclerotic plaque formation in a coronary artery.
Partial occlusion decreases coronary blood flow and leads
to symptoms of angina. Complete blockage
leads to myocardial infarction

Figure 27.1: Atheromatous plaque in coronary artery.

Answer to question two:
What initial investigations will be undertaken?

- Clinical presentation and history.
- 12 Lead ECG, to note if there are any changes and to identify region of infarction.
- BP – recorded every 15 minutes to identify how the heart is coping and to monitor for possible complications such as cardiogenic shock (Hand, 2001).
- Temperature – to monitor for complications like pericarditis but will often initially be raised due to myocardial necrosis causing an inflammatory response in the body.
- Pulse – to monitor the efficiency of the heart.
- Respiratory rate – to monitor for pulmonary oedema.
- Oxygen saturation – to monitor perfusion of oxygen.
- Continuous cardiac monitoring – to monitor heart rate and rhythm.
- Erythrocyte Sedimentation Rate – which can rise as muscle dies (Hatchett, 2001).
- Troponin-T level – a good indicator of myocardial damage (Department of Health, 2000).
- Urea and electrolyte levels – Hand (2001) considers that there is a shift in ions of potassium and sodium and as such there is the associated risk of cardiac arrhythmias. Such blood tests can also determine renal function.
- Lipid levels, random blood glucose and full blood count.
- Cardiac enzymes – there can be a raise in the creatinine kinase (CK), lactic dehydrogenase (LDH) and aspartate transaminase (AST).
- General conscious level – through observation.
- Fluid balance to monitor for heart failure and cardiogenic shock.

Answer to question three:
Explain the initial medical and nursing interventions on arrival to hospital.

Medical intervention is aimed at:

- Resuscitation of the patient
- Effective pain management
- Thrombolysis.

Resuscitation of the patient

Ranjit will be given oxygen, as he is hypoxaemic. Oxygen will be administered as prescribed via a mask. Oxygen percentage will be titrated according to oxygen saturation recordings. Vital signs will be monitored continuously to identify haemodynamic stability. Ranjit may receive other specific cardiac drugs as clinically indicated.

Effective pain management

Hatchett (2001) suggests that immediate chest pain relief is imperative. Ranjit's pain will be reassessed as he has already received diamorphine. Hand (2001) indicates this should include details regarding the pain, site, severity and duration. If pain is not relieved by using sublingual nitrates then intravenous opiates should be administered as recommended by the Department of Health (2000). Ranjit should be advised to report any chest pain immediately.

Thrombolysis

Thrombolytic therapy should be administered without delay, according to the Department of Health (2000) within an hour of the onset of symptoms. (See answer four for detailed discussion).

Nursing care

Nursing care will be based around the recording and monitoring of Ranjit's vital signs: TPR and BP and urine output. As Ranjit is initially confined to his bed he will require assistance in many of the activities of living, namely hygiene and elimination. Hand (2001) indicates that constipation should be avoided as this can put an extra strain on the heart. Ranjit's dignity should be maintained and he should be encouraged to be as self caring within the limitations of the therapeutic regime.

Often ignored for the more physiological needs, Ranjit and his family will require socio-psychological support so it is therefore important to ensure that information regarding what has happened, treatment and nursing care is explained on an ongoing basis.

Client profiles in nursing: adult & the elderly 2

Answer to question four:
Outline the role of thrombolysis and list the contraindicators and complications of its use.

Thrombolysis is given to dissolve or break down clots in the coronary arteries. Another benefit of thrombolysis is that it can limit damage to the myocardial heart muscle. The most commonly used thrombolytics are:

- Streptokinase
- Alteplase (rt-PA)
- Reteplase.

There are however contraindicators that have to be considered before thrombolysis treatment is commenced; practice areas can vary in their citeria.

- Cranial trauma (within 4 weeks)
- Previous haemorrhagic stroke
- Recent stroke
- Active peptic ulceration or other gastrointestinal blood loss
- Recent surgery
- Concurrent anticoagulation
- Severe liver disease
- Recent lumbar puncture
- Acute pancreatitis
- Uncontrolled hypertension

Hudson et al (2001)

- Received streptokinase in the last 6 months (another thrombolytic agent would have to be considered).
- Known or suspected aortic aneurysm (Hatchett, 2001)
- Recent retinal laser therapy.

Complications of the use of thrombolysis include:

- Possible allergy which can lead to an anaphylactoid reaction (streptokinase)
- Haemorrhage, either mild or severe
- Hypotension
- Reperfusion arrhythmias.

References

Department of Health (2000) National Service Framework for Coronary Heart Disease: Modern standards and service models. London: The Stationery Office.

Hand, H. (2001) Myocardial infarction: Part 1. Nursing Standard 15(36): 45–53.

Hatchett, R. (2001) Coronary Heart Disease – Part 3: The management of unstable angina, myocardial infarction and current challenges. Nursing Times 97(46): 43–46.

Hudson, I., Squire, I.B., Skehan, J.D. (2001) Coronary Care Units University Hospitals of Leicester: Management Guidelines. Leicester: Aventis.

Pearson, S. (1999) The heart, part five: coronary artery disease – 1. Nursing Times 95(47): 44–47.

Further reading

Albarran, J. (2002) The language of chest pain. Nursing Times 98(4): 38–40.

Hatchett, R., Arundale, K., Francis-Reme L. (1999) The heart, part four: basic cardiac arrhythmias. Nursing Times 95(43): 44–47.

National Institute for Clinical Excellence (2001) National Institute for Clinical Excellence (NICE) Guidelines: Prophylaxis for patients who have experienced a myocardial infarction: drug treatments, cardiac rehabilitation and dietary manipulation. London: NICE.

Pearson, S. (1999) The heart, part six: coronary heart disease – 2. Nursing Times 95(50): 42–45.

Vickers, J. (1999) The heart, part one: anatomy and physiology. Nursing Times 95(30): 42–45.

Vickers, J. (1999) The heart, part two: anatomy and physiology. Nursing Times 95(34): 46–49.

Vickers, J. (1999) The heart, part three: anatomy and physiology. Nursing Times 95(39): 46–49.

Website

www.nice.org.uk

Organ donation

Carolyn Reid

Brian Thomson is a 42-year-old chartered accountant. He is married to Sarah and they have three sons aged 12, 15 and 22 years. Whilst watching his sons playing football in the garden Brian collapsed complaining of a headache. The emergency services were called and Brian was taken to the Accident and Emergency (A & E) Department of his local hospital.

Shortly after admission to A & E Brian's Glasgow Coma Scale score dropped from 11 to 5, his pupils became dilated and unreactive to light. He was intubated and transferred to radiology for an urgent Computerised Tomography (CT) scan. This revealed a sub-arachnoid haemorrhage. Brian was admitted to the Intensive Therapy Unit for further monitoring and medical management. Intra-cranial pressure (ICP) monitoring was instituted and an arteriogram was booked. Over the course of the next few hours the medical and nursing staff found it increasingly difficult to maintain a cerebral perfusion pressure (CPP) of greater than 55 mmHg due to a labile blood pressure and increasing ICP. A further CT scan was ordered and this indicated that the extent of the bleeding had increased.

The neurosurgeon at this time spoke to Sarah and her sons and indicated that Brian was unlikely to survive due to the extent of the damage caused to the brain stem and that the medical team would be performing brain stem death tests later that evening. Although very upset the middle son indicated that his father carried an organ donor card and could this be considered as an option at this time.

Question one: How will the medical staff determine brain stem death in Brian?

30 minutes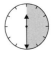

Question two: Discuss the involvement of the transplant co-ordinator in organ donation.

25 minutes

Question three: Which solid organs and tissues can be used in transplant surgery?

15 minutes

Time allowance: **70 minutes**

Answer to question one:
How will the medical staff determine brain stem death in Brian?

Before brain stem death tests can be carried out on Brian certain criteria must be met (Department of Health, 1998).

The patient must have sustained a known brain injury causing irreversible coma. Potential causes of brain stem injury include intracerebral bleed, extra-cerebral bleed (as in Brian's case), head trauma, brain tumour and a hypoxic event. Any possible causes of reversible coma need to be ruled out prior to testing (for example, administration of sedative drugs, muscle relaxants). The patient's blood chemistry should be near normal and their temperature should be greater than 35°C.

If the above criteria are met, brain stem reflexes can be assessed and these will include:

- Shining a light in the eye assesses cranial nerves II and III. The pupils will be unresponsive to light.
- Passing fine gauze or cotton wool over the cornea assesses cranial nerves V and VII. No response will be noted.
- Injecting 20 ml of ice-cold water into the external auditory canal of the tympanic membrane assesses cranial nerves III, VI and VIII. Ensure the canal is clear of residue first. The eyes should normally deviate away from the side the cold water is injected into. No eye movement will be seen.
- Applying pressure to the supra-orbital region in order to elicit a response to painful stimuli assesses cranial nerves V and VII. There will be no response.
- An attempt is made to stimulate a cough and gag reflex by manipulating the endo-tracheal tube and performing endotracheal suction assesses cranial nerves IX and X. There will be no response.
- The patient will then be disconnected from ventilatory support to assess for respiratory effort. A catheter attached to an oxygen supply will be passed down the endotracheal tube to prevent hypoxia during the procedure. The carbon dioxide level in the blood should be allowed to rise significantly in order that the chemoreceptors of central respiration will be stimulated. In brain stem death there will be no respiratory effort.
- Two medical practitioners are required to perform the brain stem death tests and are carried out twice in order to exclude observer error (Department of Health, 1998). This will usually involve the primary consultant and another doctor who has been registered at least 5 years. No medical staff with any interest in the transplant team may be involved in the brain stem testing. The time of the first set of tests is recorded as the legal time of death.

Answer to question two:
Discuss the involvement of the transplant co-ordinator in organ donation.

The Transplant Co-ordinator (TC) can be contacted at any time for information and guidance regarding organ and tissue donation. Medical or nursing staff may contact the TC to discuss the suitability of any potential donor for organ donation. Each area will have an individual approach to requesting organ donation from families. It is normal for the TC to be contacted only after brain stem death has been diagnosed and the family has agreed to organ donation following a request by the medical staff. If families have expressed an interest in organ donation prior to diagnosis of brain stem death they may be offered the opportunity to speak to the TC at an earlier stage. Some areas are now employing a collaborative approach to requesting organ donation with the involvement of the medical team and the TC (Birmingham Transplant Co-ordinators, 2002).

When contacted by the ward the TC will attend the hospital and assess the suitability of the potential donor. Current and previous medical history will be obtained from the clinical notes, medical and nursing staff. If there is any uncertainty surrounding the circumstances of the injury sustained by the patient the views of the Coroner in England and Wales or the Procurator Fiscal in Scotland will be sought. They may withhold consent to organ donation if a criminal case is a possibility.

Once the patient has been assessed as suitable for organ donation by the TC, the family will be involved in a discussion to ascertain the patient's 'lack of objection' to organ donation. They will be asked to read a document 'Keeping Transplant Safe'. This document screens the potential donor's social history. The family is made aware that further blood tests are necessary before donation can proceed. These include screening for hepatitis and human immuno deficiency virus (HIV). A request is made to contact the patient's GP to further investigate their medical history.

When the TC completes all necessary documentation, a call is made to UK Transplant (UKT) in Bristol. UKT hold all the records of patients awaiting a transplant. They will inform the TC if there are any patients waiting urgently for a transplant. These patients will be offered the organs first. Local retrieval teams will then be contacted and arrangements will be made for their arrival in the hospital and a suitable theatre time will be set. The care of the patient on the ward continues with an emphasis on preserving organ function prior to the donation. The TC will follow the patient to theatre and following completion of the surgical procedure will assist the theatre staff in performing last offices.

The TC will follow up recipient patients. A follow-up letter can be sent to the donor family if requested updating them on the progress of the recipients.

Organ donation is now occurring in non-heart beating donors (Lewis & Valerius, 1999). Several centers in England are running a programme whereby families can be approached when a patient is near death, perhaps following a stroke. A transplant team will attend the patient shortly after death to retrieve the kidneys.

There are age limits specific to each organ, but these are constantly being reviewed so no patient should be excluded because of their age before checking with the TC. Corneas can be retrieved from birth to 100 years of age.

Question three: Describe the post-operative care that Mr Ahmed will require for the first 48 hours, giving rationale for your actions.

25 minutes

Time allowance: **55 minutes**

Answer to question one:
What is meant by the term aneurysm?

An aneurysm can be defined as a local dilatation of a blood vessel (the Greek word aneurysm means a 'widening'). The area of the vessel wall becomes progressively weaker as the aneurysm gradually enlarges, and the risk of spontaneous rupture increases (Bick, 2000).

Answer to question two:
List the investigations that will be carried out on Mr Ahmed prior to surgery.

Several tests are available to confirm the diagnosis and to classify its location:

- Spinal computerised tomography is useful for sizing the aneurysm.
- Magnetic resonance imaging is able to identify the size and location.
- Transoesophageal echocardiography is exceedingly accurate and can provide additional information on ventricular function, aortic valve competency and left main coronary artery patency (Blanchard et al, 1994).
- A range of blood tests: a full blood count, urea and electrolytes, creatinine clearance and blood lipids are taken to obtain baseline values and identify any problems such as renal damage or anaemia.
- Chest X-ray.
- Clotting studies.

Answer to question three:
Describe the post-operative care that Mr Ahmed will require for the first 48 hours, giving rationale for your actions.

On return from operation, Mr Ahmed will have his observations recorded. These will include:

- Blood pressure and pulse will be recorded continuously via an arterial line and should be documented every 15 minutes for the first hour (Collins, 2001). Hypertension can cause bleeding around the graft site and lead to rupture of the graft. Hypotension may indicate haemorrhage and shock.
- Mechanical ventilation – Mr Ahmed will be sedated, paralysed and ventilated to maintain adequate perfusion. When Mr Ahmed is able to maintain spontaneous respiration he will be extubated. Post extubation he will be nursed in an upright position to promote lung expansion, and ensure that deep breathing and chest physiotherapy is maintained (Herbert, 1997). Oxygen as prescribed will be administered to prevent hypoxia.
- Temperature – initially he will be peripherally cold – there is a gradual warming of peripheries until patient is normothermic: a rise in temperature will indicate infection at the graft site/wound site. An unnoticed infected graft will prolong the patient's stay in hospital and cause more suffering.
- Conscious level – there is an increased risk of stroke as clots are dislodged and new ones may be formed. It may be difficult to assess the risk of such a complication whilst the patient is mechanically ventilated.
- Central venous pressure (CVP) – to monitor the cardiovascular status. A low CVP reading and a low urine output may indicate reduced blood volume due to either haemorrhage or dehydration. Intravenous fluids, whole blood or plasma protein substitute will be required to correct the deficit (see Case 20).
- A low urine output and a high CVP may indicate renal shutdown.
- Tissue perfusion of the lower limbs can be monitored by observing for the presence of pedal pulses, warmth, movement and sensitivity. It should be noted that limb cyanosis may be more difficult to detect because of the dark skin colour of the patient. A change may indicate that the graft is blocked and this will necessitate emergency surgery to unblock the graft.
- Nil by mouth (NBM) – Mr Ahmed will remain NBM until bowel sound returns and there is no nausea or sickness, therefore a nasogastric tube may be inserted for the initial post-operative period. Mr Ahmed will start taking sips of water and the volume is gradually increased as tolerated until a light diet can be taken.
- Fluid and hydration – intravenous infusions will continue until Mr Ahmed is able to take oral fluids to maintain his own hydration.
- Pain management – good pain control is essential. Assess Mr Ahmed's pain frequently and administer analgesics as prescribed. Monitor their effectiveness and side effects.

- Wound – a large transverse wound will be present. The wound will be covered and the dressing should be observed for any leakage.
- Mobilisation – Mr Ahmed should be mobilised as soon as possible. He should be encouraged to exercise his legs gently and may be helped to get out of bed the next day. As mobility is limited complications of immobility should be observed for.
- Mr Ahmed will require assistance with his physical needs such as hygiene, mouth care and elimination. His psychological well being should not be forgotten and he and his family should be kept well informed of what is happening.

References

Bick, C. (2000) Abdominal aortic aneurysm repair. Nursing Standard 15(3): 47–52.

Blanchard, D.G., Kimura, B.J., Diltrich, H.C. et al (1994) Transoesophageal echocardiography of the aorta. Journal of American Medical Association 272: 546–551.

Collins, F. (2001) Abdominal Aortic Aneurysm Repair. In: Murray, S. Vascular Disease: Nursing and Management. London: Whurr Publishers.

Herbert, L. (1997) Caring for the Vascular Patient. New York: Churchill Livingstone.

Chronic obstructive pulmonary disease

Kim Leong

Mr Paul Clayton is a 75-year-old widower. He has two grown up children. His eldest daughter lives locally. His son, a businessman lives in London.

Paul lives in a semi-detached house. He is a heavy smoker, smoking cigarettes for the past 60 years. He relies on his daughter to do his shopping and other chores, as these can be exhausting for him. He enjoyed gardening, but increasingly he has been unable to do such physical work.

Paul has been suffering from chronic obstructive pulmonary disease (COPD) for a number of years. One week ago he visited his General Practitioner (GP) because of increasing dyspnoea and he was prescribed a course of antibiotics for a chest infection.

However, Paul's condition has continued to deteriorate, he has become breathless at rest and he is expectorating thin, purulent, copious sputum. His daughter called for an ambulance and he was admitted to a Medical Admissions Unit. After initial investigations, Paul was diagnosed as having a severe chest infection, which was not responding to initial treatment prescribed by the GP.

Question one: What is COPD?

5 minutes

Question two: What pathophysiological changes occur in COPD?

10 minutes

Question three: What interventions will Paul require on arrival to the Medical Admissions Unit?

30 minutes

Question four: What measures can be taken to minimise further exacerbations caused by chest infections?

15 minutes

Time allowance: **60 minutes**

Answer to question one:
What is COPD?

COPD is an umbrella term used to describe a range of lung conditions and includes: chronic bronchitis, chronic asthma and emphysema. It is defined by the British Thoracic Society (BTS) as a chronic slowly progressing disorder characterised by airway obstruction which does not change markedly over several months (BTS, 1997).

* Chronic bronchitis can be defined as 'the presence of a chronic cough and sputum production for at least three months on two consecutive years in the absence of other diseases recognised to cause sputum production'. (Fehrenbach, 1998, 771)
* Chronic asthma – airflow obstruction through narrowing of the bronchioles.
* Emphysema is the permanent abnormal enlargement of the air spaces due to destruction of alveolar walls (See Fig. 30.1 & 30. 2).

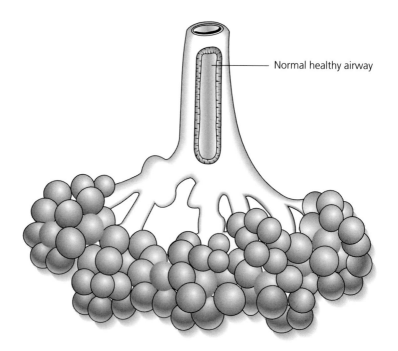

Normal healthy airway

Figure 30.1: Normal airway.

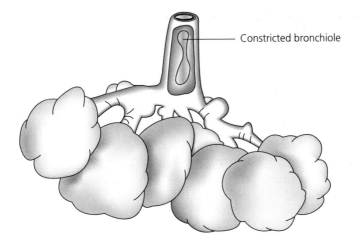

Constricted bronchiole

Figure 30.2: Constricted bronchiole and hyper-inflated alveoli in emphysema.

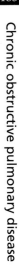

Answer to question two:
What pathophysiological changes occur in COPD?

Chronic bronchitis

There is chronic inflammation of the mucus membrane of the tracheo-bronchial tree. As a result of the inflammation and irritation of the tracheo-bronchial tree, there is hypertrophy of the mucus glands. The number of goblet cells is increased and the ciliated epithelia are paralysed (Walsh, 1997). The impaired ciliary movement will lead to mucus stasis and infections as a consequence. This mucus plugging causes the respiratory airways to be narrowed. The narrowed lumen will lead to airflow limitations and causes the person to experience wheeziness and breathlessness. The person may become weak, cyanosed and disorientated due to lack of oxygen.

Emphysema

The narrowed lumen in the respiratory tree causes the air pressure to rise. This results in the rupture of the alveoli (bullae). The loss of air sacs leads to a decrease in the surface area for gaseous exchange. Consequently, there is a decrease in the volume of oxygen in each intake of breath and the person needs to breathe faster in order to compensate.

The patient tends to hunch over in order to help the accessory muscles of respiration to function effectively. The patient also develops a pattern of pursed lip breathing, which causes him to slow the rate at which breath is expired, preventing pressure drops that may cause airways to collapse.

Chronic asthma

In this condition there is irreversible bronchoconstriction resulting in persistent symptoms of wheeze and dyspnoea.

Answer to question three:
What interventions will Paul require on arrival to the Medical Admissions Unit?

The symptoms of chronic bronchitis and emphysema can vary from one patient to another, so accurate assessment is imperative.

Medical interventions

• Pharmacological intervention

The most common method of treating a patient with an exacerbation of chronic bronchitis and emphysema is the administration of bronchodilators via a nebuliser. Nebulisation is a method of turning a drug or solution into a mist, which is inhaled directly into the airways. The most common nebulised drugs are bronchodilators. The current bronchodilator used is ipratropium bromide, which is an anticholinergic drug (Abrams, 2001). Ventolin, a beta2 agonist is also used for adequate bronchodilatation.

Steroids such as hydrocortisone (intravenously) or prednisolone (orally) can also be administered to reduce the inflammation in the airways. Initially, a broad-spectrum antibiotic may be administered. An appropriate antibiotic can be administered when the result of the culture and sensitivity is known.

Paul should be given a low percentage of prescribed oxygen. In a healthy person, the carbon dioxide levels (pCO_2) in the blood stimulates the respiratory centre. In contrast, a person with chronic bronchitis and emphysema responds to a relatively low level of oxygen and it is this mechanism that drives him to breathe (hypoxic drive).

• Investigations

A number of investigations will be carried ⸱scertain the presence or severity of COPD; these will include:
Spirometry – a forced expiratory volume ⸱⸱cate the severity of the COPD.
Chest X-ray – used to diagnose emphys⸢ conditions.
Arterial blood gases – will indicate hy⸤
Computerised tomography scan – to ⸤
Echocardiogram – to assess heart fun⸤
Electrocardiogram – to identify isch⸤
Haematology and biochemistry – polycythaemia.
Microbiology – sputum specimen⸤

• Specific nursing intervention

Paul's comfort should be may⸤ encouraged to comply with b⸤ should be made available a⸤ physiotherapist may teach⸤

Patients who experience difficulty in breathing are often anxious and distressed. Paul should be given appropriate information, support and reassurance. When explaining any treatment and procedures carried out, it is important that information is given slowly because an anxious patient or relative cannot focus or retain information readily. Paul may be experiencing pain both from the chest infection and as a consequence of using his accessory muscles when breathing. Analgesics will be given to Paul to manage his pain. Paul's vital signs should be monitored closely for respiratory depression.

Answer to question four:
What measures can be taken to minimise further exacerbations caused by chest infections?

- Smoking

The primary cause of chronic bronchitis and emphysema is due to a long-term smoking habit (Groer, 2001). The deterioration of this condition can be prevented even though the emphysematous nature of the disease is not reversible. Cessation of smoking can halt the deterioration of this condition. It can therefore make a difference to the patient's quality of life, morbidity and mortality. A smoking cessation pack can be obtained from the local health promotion unit. Paul should be advised to stop smoking.

- Prevention of infection

Since the primary cause of the exacerbation of chronic bronchitis and emphysema is due to an infection, measures must be taken to halt this. Paul must be advised to try to avoid overcrowding, especially to avoid being in the same room with people who have infections. He should be offered the influenza vaccination. He must be reminded of the importance of completing his antibiotic in order to avoid developing resistant organisms.

- Oxygen therapy at home

Paul may be assessed for oxygen therapy at home. If oxygen therapy is appropriate, he must then be given advice on the correct percentage of oxygen in order to prevent complications and safety.

- Pulmonary and nutritional rehabilitation

Paul must be given advice on proper breathing exercises, sleep strategies and the avoidance of exercises that may compromise his cardiopulmonary system. He should be taught how to recognise the early signs and symptoms of a deterioration in his condition.

He must be given advice on diet, which should be well balanced, containing the right proportion of carbohydrate, proteins, fats, water, minerals, vitamins and fibres (Dudek, 2001).

- Compliance

Compliance is important especially because Paul will have to take medications on an ongoing basis to prevent further exacerbation of his condition. Paul's compliance should be evaluated on a regular basis.

References

Abrams, A.C. (2001) Clinical Drug Therapy: Rationales for Nursing Practice. New York: Lippincott.

British Thoracic Society (1997) Guidelines for the management of COPD. Thorax 52(55): S1–S32.

Dudek, S.G. (2001) Nutrition Essentials for Nursing Practice. (4th ed.). New York: Lippincott.

Client profiles in nursing: adult & the elderly 2

Fehrenbach, C. (1998) Chronic obstructive pulmonary disease. Professional Nurse 13(11): 771–777.

Groer, M. (2001) Advanced Pathophysiology: Application to Clinical Practice. New York: Lippincott.

Walsh, M. (1997) Watson's Clinical Nursing & Related Science. (5th ed.). London: Bailliere Tindall.

Further reading

Paradisco, C. (1999) Lippincott's Review Series: The Ideal Study Aid. Here's Why .... Pathophysiology. (2nd ed.). New York: Lippincott.

Exploring the grandparent(s) role

Chris Buswell

Mrs Gertrude Wade is a 62-year-old widow, learning to live with the effects of rheumatoid arthritis. She retired early from her part time job as a florist due to painful joints and the increasing pain in her hands which affected her job. Soon after retiring, her daughter, Sonia, asked Mrs Wade if she would look after her first baby Scott, while she went out to work. Mrs Wade was glad to do this to help support Sonia, and also to feel she was contributing to Scott's development. Mrs Wade feels that Scott has become a confident youngster and feels a sense of pride that she contributed to his upbringing. She is particularly proud of the way Scott helps her around the house when he comes to visit.

Sonia is visiting her mother with Scott, and 6 month old Patrick.

'Now that Scott is settled at school I thought I'd apply for my old job in the office. I've heard the lady who replaced me is leaving and my former manager phoned me up the other day and said I really should apply for it,' said Sonia to her mother.

'That sounds great Sonia, but what about baby Patrick? I know you've missed going to work, but I thought Neil's promotion and pay rise was seeing you all alright. Wouldn't you be better off staying at home and securing the future of your children?'

'Oh mum I miss work and all my friends. I miss the banter with the girls and the challenge of work. As much as I love my children I need to develop myself. I was hoping you'd look after Patrick, like you did Scott. Scott's turned into such a lovely, helpful boy. I'm sure that's down to you. Couldn't you look after Patrick too, after all Scott will be at school, and I'll get time off during the holidays. Please say you will mum,' asked Sonia as she looked at her mother hopefully.

'Oh Sonia,' sighed her mother, 'I'd hoped you wouldn't ask me that. You see I'm not as able as I was when I looked after Scott. I really loved looking after Scott. He's such a lovely boy, and so is Patrick. Scott made me feel young again, almost like a second parent-hood, although not with your dear dad here to enjoy it. If only dad was still alive I'd say yes straight away, but on my own I can't cope with Patrick. Look at my hands now Sonia, see how deformed and painful they are,' said Mrs Wade as she held her hands up in the air.

'I know your arthritis is getting worse and you find it difficult to do certain things, but Patrick will be no trouble,' replied Sonia.

'For Patrick's safety I have to say no Sonia. I'd never be able to open those tiny baby food jars or change a small nappy with these clumsy hands, not even with the gadgets your Neil bought me. I'd feel awful if something happened because I was too weak or wasn't able to do something. It's not fair on me nor Patrick. As helpful as Scott is even he can't help me with a baby, especially as he'll be at school and I'll be on my own. I can still baby sit at night when they're safely tucked up in bed, and I'll still collect Scott from school for you and walk him home. I'm sorry Sonia I just can't look after Patrick full time like I did Scott, I'm just not up to it. But let me do other things to help, you know I love seeing my grandchildren.'

Question one: Discuss grandparenthood and the role that grandparents play in the development of their grandchildren.

Time allowance: **1 hour**

Answer to question one:
Discuss grandparenthood and the role that grandparents play in the development of their grandchildren.

One of the most important roles of some elderly people is their role as grandparent. The support they offer their children and their children's children should not be underestimated. Nor should the experience of being a grandparent be forgotten. Grandparents can obtain enjoyment, affection and a sense of purpose through their grandchildren who may provide a new interest and meaning to life (Eliopoulos, 1993). In turn grandparents may receive unconditional love and attention from their grandchildren which continue into their grandchildren's adulthood (Eliopoulos, 1993).

Grandparents should not be seen as the older old now, as they can often be in their forties or fifties (Heath & Schofield, 1999). Therefore when grandparenting is discussed it also encompasses great grandparents and possibly even great, great grandparents.

Traditionally, in the extended family, grandparents played an active role in child care so that they in turn would feel secure knowing that the family unit would care for them when they had increased requirements for assistance (Eliopoulos, 1993). However now that families may move, perhaps to secure better jobs, the family structure is changing (Eliopoulos, 1993).

Figure 31.1 displays topics for discussion based on the work of American psychologist Helen Kivnick (1982) whose work revealed the many roles that grandparents may fulfill. Grandparents often have good relationships with their grandchildren and may have a knowledge and understanding of issues faced by their grandchildren which allows them to act as health educators (Heath & Schofield, 1999). In addition to these roles many grandparents are taking on part time child care responsibilities for their grandchildren, particularly for divorced or single parent children (Heath & Schofield, 1999), perhaps through love, a sense of obligation or a belief in traditional values (Davidhizar, Bechtel & Woodring, 2000; Dowdell & Sherwen, 1998). Other grandparents may take on full time care for their grandchildren after the death of their own children and their spouses (Davidhizar, Bechtel & Woodring, 2000). Other grandparents may have to care for their grandchildren full time due to parents' drug

---

- Grandparents play a central role in the upbringing of their grandchildren.
- Grandparents promote a sense of family history.
- Through their grandchildren, grandparents are able to relive their past.
- Grandparents may be seen by their grandchildren as esteemed elders.
- Grandparents may indulge their grandchildren.

(Kivnick, 1982)

Figure 31.1: Mrs Gertrude Wade, grandparenthood.

addictions, prison sentences and the growing problem of HIV and AIDS (Dowdell & Sherwen, 1998).

Some grandparents, like Mrs Wade when she cared for Scott, may attain a sense of purpose in their new role (Thompson, Itzin & Abendstern, 1991). Some children may feel that they have missed out from not having grandparents (Thompson, Itzin & Abendstern, 1991). Children who grow up within a close relationship with their grandparents are more likely to have more positive attitudes towards older people (Heath & Schofield, 1999).

Other authors describe the negative effects of caring for or raising grand-children full time. These include financial stress, diminished marital satisfaction, cramped living conditions, social isolation, role restriction, retiring earlier to devote time to grandchildren, all of which could lead to grandparents being at risk of social isolation and developing mental and emotional problems (Davidhizar, Bechtel & Woodring, 2000; Dowdell & Sherwen, 1998). Such problems may be hindered by changing attitudes of society on how to bring up children compared to the days when grandparents were parents themselves, and the scarce resources and advice for grandparents (Davidhizar, Bechtel & Woodring, 2000). Modern day problems such as children exposed to drugs, alcohol, cyberporn and child prostitution may bring fresh challenges to grandparents (Davidhizar, Bechtel & Woodring, 2000; Dowdell & Sherwen, 1998). Ageing changes and changing health status may also affect grandparents caring for grandchildren (Dowdell & Sherwen, 1998). Some grandparents may put the needs of their grandchildren before their own health care needs (Davidhizar, Bechtel & Woodring, 2000).

However some grandparents may welcome full time child care again. Some find it brings a positive effect to their relationships with their spouse due to the increased communication and the fresh challenge of new life goals (Davidhizar, Bechtel & Woodring, 2000). Others feel a sense of pride at keeping a traditional family unit together (Caliandro & Hughes, 1998).

References

Caliandro, G., Hughes, C. (1998) The experience of being a grandmother who is the primary care giver for her HIV positive grandchild. Nursing Research 47(2): 107–113.

Davidhizar, R., Bechtel, G.A., Woodring, B.C. (2000) The changing role of grandparenthood. Journal of Gerontological Nursing 26(1): 24–29.

Dowdell, E.B., Sherwen, L.N. (1998) Grandmothers who raise grandchildren: a cross-generational challenge to caregivers. Journal of Gerontological Nursing 24(5): 8–13.

Eliopoulos, C. (1993) Gerontological Nursing. (3rd ed.). Philadelphia: J.B. Lippincott Company.

Heath, H., Schofield, I. (1999) (Eds) Healthy Ageing: Nursing Older People. London: Mosby.

Kivnick, H. (1982) Grandparenthood: An overview of meaning and mental health. Gerontologist 22, 59 cited in: Heath, H., Schofield, I. (1999) (Eds) Healthy Ageing: Nursing Older People. London: Mosby.

Thompson, P., Itzin, C., Abendstern, M. (1991) I Don't Feel Old. Oxford: Oxford University Press cited in: Heath, H., Schofield, I. (1999) (Eds) Healthy Ageing: Nursing Older People. London: Mosby.

Liver failure

Sam Parboteeah

Mrs Eileen Bishop is 46 years old and is married to Geoffrey. They have three children aged 16, 18 and 21 years, all still living at home. Eileen is the manager of the family catering business and works very long hours. She also travels a lot and often spends time away from home. She had been a social drinker consuming about 16 units of alcohol per week after returning from work in the evenings. However, over the recent months her alcohol consumption has increased to 40 units per week as she is feeling increasingly tired, with the pressure of work and sharing the household responsibilites.

Eileen has found it difficult to maintain her concentration at work and there have been complaints about her drinking from other members of the family. Eileen has complained of nausea and vomiting and reluctantly accepts her husband's advice to see her General Practitioner (GP).

Eileen admits to her GP about the increase in her alcohol consumption of the last few months. A physical examination indicates the presence of an enlarged tender liver. Liver function tests confirm that Eileen has developed alcoholic hepatitis and she is advised to rest from work and to abstain from drinking alcohol. She is admitted to a medical ward with acute pain.

Question one: Describe the macroscopic structure of the liver and show the dual blood supply of the liver.

20 minutes

Question two: Describe the functions of the liver.

20 minutes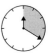

Question three: List the signs and symptoms of alcoholic hepatitis.

15 minutes

Question four: Discuss the nursing and medical care that Eileen will require whilst in hospital.

25 minutes

Time allowance: **80 minutes**

Answer to question one:
Describe the macroscopic structure of the liver and show the dual blood supply of the liver.

The liver is the largest organ in the body and in an adult it weighs between 1–2.3 kg (Wilson & Waugh, 1996). It is located in the upper part of the abdominal cavity occupying the greater part of the right hypochondriac region and extending into the left hypochondriac region. The liver is enclosed in a thin capsule and incompletely covered by a layer of peritoneum. The liver has four lobes: right lobe (the largest), a smaller wedge shaped left lobe, the other two the caudate and quadrate lobes are areas on the posterior surface (Fig. 32.1).

The hepatic artery and the portal vein take blood to the liver. The hepatic artery contributes only one fifth to one third of the supply and the rest of the supply is brought by the portal vein. The blood supply delivered via the portal vein comes from the venous drainage of most of the gastrointestinal tract (Fig. 32.2) and is rich in digested nutrients and is partially deoxygenated (Rutishauser, 1994).

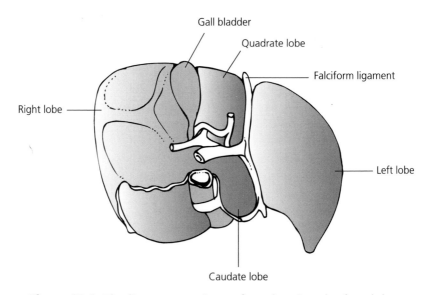

Figure 32.1: The liver – posterior surface showing the four lobes.

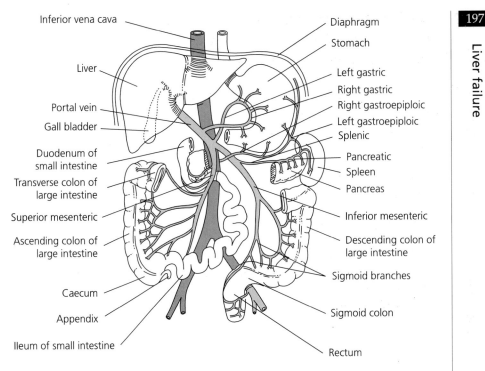

Figure 32.2: Hepatic portal circulation.

Answer to question two:
Describe the functions of the liver.

The functions of the liver can be divided into four main categories:

• Destruction
• Heat
• Synthesis
• Storage.

Destruction

1. The liver is responsible for the deamination of proteins (the removal of the amine group) and for converting into ammonia. The ammonia is then converted to urea which is then excreted in the urine. This is performed exclusively by the liver. Ammonia cannot be excreted as such and if not converted to urea it accumulates in the blood causing confusion, drowsiness and coma.
2. Nucleic acids are broken down and converted to uric acid.
3. Triglycerides can be broken down by the liver lipase to fatty acids and glycerol. Fatty acids can be partly metabolised in the liver to ketones which can then be fully oxidised by the other tissues of the body for energy.
4. Kupffer cells are specialised cells of the immune system and phagocytose foreign particles.
5. The liver removes poisons or potential poisons (for example, drugs). Some substances are destroyed, others are conjugated (joined with something else to make them harmless). These substances are then excreted via the bile and urine.
6. The liver also destroys worn out red cells.
7. The liver eliminates some hormones (for example, cortisol, oestrogen, testosterone, anti-diuretic hormone).

Heat

The liver is an important heat producing organ in the body. In liver failure, the patient becomes hypothermic.

Synthesis

1. Bile salts are manufactured in the liver.
2. Bilirubin is conjugated in the liver, rendering it water soluble. In liver failure there may be accumulation of bilirubin resulting in jaundice.
3. Plasma proteins (albumin, globulins, clotting factors, vitamin K) are produced in the liver.
4. The liver produces heparin and antibodies.

5. The liver can also convert one amino acid to another by the process of transamination.
6. The liver is able to convert its stored glycogen to glucose (glycogenolysis) and to convert amino acids, lactic acid into glycogen and glucose (gluconeogenesis).

Storage

The liver stores small amount of glucose (glycogen), fat, amino acids, vitamins A, D and K, and substances required for erythropoesis (formation of red blood cells).

Answer to question three:
List the signs and symptoms of alcoholic hepatitis.

The signs and symptoms which a patient may present are varied and include:

- Anorexia
- Vomiting
- Jaundice
- Fever
- Confusion, delirium and tremor
- Spider naevi
- Large liver
- Liver function test may show an increased level of transferase.

Answer to question four:
Discuss the nursing and medical care that Eileen will require whilst in hospital.

The main aim of medical intervention is to control Eileen's symptoms, minimise the risk of potential complications and support her to abstain from alcohol abuse. Management will include:

- Pain relief – Eileen's pain could be relieved by placing her into a comfortable position and the administration of prescribed analgesics (these should be administered with precaution to avoid hepatotoxic effects). Pain caused by pruritis can be relieved by the application of soothing lotions (calamine lotion) and anti-histamines.
- Nutritional support – Eileen should be encouraged to take a diet rich in protein (Tait, 1995) and low salt to reduce oedema (Miller et al, 1994).
- Fluid restriction – if ascites is present then fluids may be restricted and Eileen's blood urea, electrolytes and biochemistry will be monitored. To identify if fluid is being retained Eileen should be weighed daily.
- Observation of potential complications – Eileen will be observed for any bruising or bleeding. Signs and symptoms of liver encephalopathy will be observed for as well as the recording and reporting of all vital signs including the level of consciousness and behaviour changes.
- Minimising anxiety – this may be due to fear of the outcome of the disease and the threat to the family business. She should be encouraged to ask questions and verbalise her fears. Staff should also explain all procedures and give information as necessary.
- Loss of self concept – as a result of her admission to hospital, Eileen may feel that her role in the business may be affected as would her body image and self esteem. The ward should provide an environment in which a trusting relationship can develop and staff should be non judgemental in their attitudes to her. Eileen may be referred to a counsellor for additional help.
- Potential complications of immobility – Eileen's mobility may be limited. A risk assessment should be undertaken and intervention planned accordingly.
- Eileen may be craving for alcohol. Staff should handle the situation sensitively by listening to Eileen, observing her behaviour and reassuring her as much as possible. In the acute stages, she may receive medication to control her symptoms.

References

Miller, R., Howie, E., Murchie, M. (1994) The gastrointestinal system: liver and bilary tract. In: Alexander, M. et al. Nursing Practice Hospital and Home: The Adult. Edinburgh: Churchill Livingstone.

Rutishauser, S. (1994) Physiology and Anatomy: A Basis for Nursing and Health Care. Edinburgh: Churchill Livingstone.

Tait, D.J. (1995) Care implications of disorders of thought and perception. In: Peattie, P.I., Walker, S. Understanding Nursing Care. Edinburgh: Churchill Livingstone.

Wilson, K.J.W., Waugh, A. (1996) Ross and Wilson – Anatomy and Physiology in Health and Illness. New York: Churchill Livingstone.

Useful address

Alcoholics Anonymous
PO Box 1
Stonebow House
Stonebow
York YO1 7NJ
Tel: 01904 644026

Arterial surgery

Kim Leong

Mr Jim Jabberskowski, is a 82-year-old widower who lives in a terraced house in the middle of an industrial city.

Originally born in Poland, he came to the United Kingdom after the Second World War. Since the death of his wife, 10 years ago, he has become somewhat isolated with no immediate family in the country.

Jim likes doing the daily crossword and puzzles in the newspaper. He also enjoys going occasionally to the Polish Club. He has two dogs and he walks them daily in the local park.

Increasingly he is finding it more difficult to walk. He is stopping more frequently because he is getting pain in his left leg which is relieved after a period of rest. He has found it useful to use a walking stick for support.

He is awaiting surgery to improve his circulation.

Question one: What is intermittent claudication?

5 minutes

Question two: What are the underlying pathophysiological changes and clinical features that Mr Jabberskowski may exhibit?

15 minutes

Question three: What investigations are Mr Jabberskowski likely to have to confirm the diagnosis?

10 minutes

Question four: Explain what is a femoro-popliteal bypass and how the graft function should be monitored.

15 minutes

Question five: What advice would you give on Mr Jabberskowski's discharge?

15 minutes

Time allowance: **60 minutes**

Answer to question one:
What is intermittent claudication?

Intermittent claudication, sometimes known as 'exercise pain' is the most common symptom in peripheral arterial disease. During the exercise of a limb in a healthy individual, a rapid increase in blood supply normally occurs. When there is narrowing or obstruction of arteries, this increase in blood supply cannot occur and the patient experiences pain as a result of the build up of lactic acid which restricts mobility.

Answer to question two:
What are the underlying pathophysiological changes and clinical features that Mr Jabberskowski may exhibit?

Due to the narrowing of the femoral artery there is a diminished blood supply to his affected leg. The left foot will be affected first because it is furthest away from the femoral artery (Paradisco, 1999). The toe or toes will appear cold and pale or blue. The red-purple discolouration is a sign of arterial insufficiency. There is also parasthesia, a decreased sensation in the extremities sometimes described as tingling or numbing. It is very difficult to feel the pulse below the point of narrowed artery. If there is a total blockage, the pulse below the point of blockage will not be palpable. Another sign that can easily be observed is the wasting of the calf muscle compared to the good leg.

Answer to question three:
What investigations are Mr Jabberskowski likely to have to confirm the diagnosis?

A Doppler test (an ultrasonic device) is used to detect the quality of blood flow and if there is a blockage in the artery.

Mr Jabberskowski should also have a femoral arteriogram. The radiologist (Hutton, 1993) carries out this procedure by puncturing the femoral artery. A radio-opaque dye is then introduced in the artery. A series of X-rays will then be taken to show the location of the stricture or obstruction in the affected artery. It is very important that the nurse applies pressure to the puncture site before a pressure bandage is secured in place. This is carried out to prevent any haemorrhage from the puncture site.

Answer to question four:
Explain what is a femoro-popliteal bypass and how the graft function should be monitored.

It is a procedure that attempts to bypass the obstruction and therefore improve the supply of blood to the ischaemic leg.

There are two possible types of graft that can be used:

- A length of the saphenous vein can be used as a graft (autograft ensures there is no future rejection). One end of the saphenous vein is anastamosed above the blockage and the other below the blockage (Fig. 33.1).
- Synthetic grafts may be used if no satisfactory vein is available.

Graft function can be monitored by:

- Observing the colour, movement and sensation of the left leg
- Presence of pedal pulse
- Reporting of pain in left leg
- Signs of numbness and tingling.

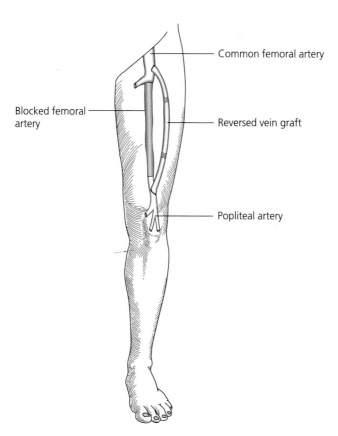

Common femoral artery

Blocked femoral artery

Reversed vein graft

Popliteal artery

Figure 33.1: Femoro-popliteal bypass.

Answer to question five:
What advice would you give on Mr Jabberskowski's discharge?

Mr Jabberskowski should be advised to stop smoking and provided with appropriate information and support, since this is one of the major causes of atherosclerosis resulting in peripheral vascular disease.

He should also be encouraged to take a low fat diet. Therefore, referral to a dietician should be considered. Good nutrition is essential to promote wound healing and prevent tissue breakdown.

Mr Jabberskowski must be encouraged to mobilise so that his general circulation will increase. Increased circulation will help to prevent deep vein thrombosis and pulmonary embolism (Lakhani et al, 1993). Mobilisation will not only give him a sense of independence but also well being, self-worth, an increase of self-esteem, morale and confidence. As a result of mobilisation his appetite will increase, and pressure sores can also be prevented.

Mr Jabberskowski should be encouraged to wear warm clothing in cold weather conditions as low temperatures cause vasoconstriction and reduction of blood flow that may damage the tissues in the toes (Walsh, 1997). He should be advised to take a warm drink and seek a warm environment. At night he should be advised to wear warm socks to keep the feet warm and avoid using direct heat as this may damage his skin. Jim should be extra vigilant in caring for his feet.

Following discussion with Jim, a referral may be made to social services and the primary healthcare team so support is available to him on discharge. Ryan (1994) points out that the smooth transition from hospital to home is essential as any unmet needs can undo most of the previous progress.

References

Hutton, A.R. (1993) An Introduction to Medical Terminology: A Self-Teaching Package. London: Churchill Livingstone.

Lakhani, S.R., Dilly, S.A., Finlayson, C.J. (1993) Basic Pathology: An Introduction to the Mechanisms of Disease. London: Edward Arnold.

Paradisco, C. (1999) Lippincott's Review Series: The Ideal Study Aid. Here's Why… . Pathophysiology. (2nd ed.). New York: Lippincott.

Ryan, A. (1994) Improving discharge planning. Nursing Times 90(20): 33–34.

Walsh, M. (1997) Watson's Clinical Nursing & Related Science. (5th ed.). London: Bailliere Tindall.

Further reading

Abrams, A.C. (2001) Clinical Drug Therapy: Rationales for Nursing Practice. New York: Lippincott.

Hinchliff, S.M., Montague, S.E., Watson, R. (1996) Physiology for Nursing Practice. (2nd ed.). London: Bailliere Tindall.

Total gastrectomy

Liz Shears & Julia Ball

Vijay Singh, is a 64-year-old Asian gentleman who emigrated to England over 40 years ago. He is married and they have two sons and two daughters and have built up a thriving news agency business. All his children are married and live locally, providing good family support. His eldest son helps Vijay run the news agency. His social life mainly revolves around his family. He takes a vegetarian diet, does not drink alcohol and smokes about 30 cigarettes a day.

Vijay developed dyspepsia about a year ago, for which he self medicated with antacid tablets. In the last month he has experienced regurgitation of food and occasional vomiting following meals with a resulting weight loss and anorexia. His General Practitioner (GP) sent Vijay for an endoscopy during which a lesion in his stomach was biopsied. The result of this confirmed a diagnosis of carcinoma of the stomach. Following a hospital outpatient appointment it is arranged that Vijay will be admitted for a total gastrectomy.

As part of his pre-operative preparation Vijay had blood samples taken to assess liver function, urea and electrolytes and a full blood count. His blood was also cross matched for transfusion postoperatively. Other tests included a chest X-ray and electrocardiogram.

During this period he was seen by the physiotherapist, who taught him deep breathing exercises whilst advising him to stop smoking pre operatively. The dietician undertook a nutritional assessment which indicated that whilst he had lost some weight as a result of his anorexia he did not require nutritional supplements pre operatively. At this stage it was also discussed with Vijay the dietary requirements he would require after surgery. A routine urinalysis was undertaken and a pressure ulcer risk assessment tool used to identify a baseline and determine if he required additional care to prevent tissue damage.

His pre-operative preparation included giving Vijay and his family information about his operation and post-operative period. A visit to the high dependency area to which Vijay would go following surgery was also arranged for all the family in an attempt to allay any anxieties they may have and to make the area more familiar to them.

His immediate preparation for surgery included pre-operative fasting, taking a shower and skin preparation as per local policy. He was fitted with anti embolism stockings and commenced injections of low molecular heparin. Following completion of his theatre check list he was given prescribed premedication and taken to the operating theatre.

Upon his return to the high dependency area his operating notes indicated that Vijay had a total gastrectomy and that his liver was clear of metastases. His pain was controlled by epidural analgesia.

Question one: Explain what observations need to be done in relation to the management of his epidural analgesia.

20 minutes

Question two: Identify the nursing care that Vijay will need during the first 48 hours after his return from theatre.

40 minutes

Question three: What advice and help may be given to Vijay by the multi disciplinary team to prepare Vijay for his discharge home?

15 minutes

Time allowance: **75 minutes**

Answer to question one:
Explain what observations need to be done in relation to the management of his epidural analgesia.

Local policy will reflect the nature and frequency of patient observations that need to be carried out in order that the development of complications may be detected early and to monitor the effectiveness of the epidural analgesia. Observations include:

- Blood pressure
- Respiratory assessment
- Sedation score
- Oxygen saturation rate.

Observations are recorded every 15 minutes for the first hour after insertion of the epidural catheter, hourly then onwards for the next 24 hours and then 4 hourly. Each time a bag is changed, the vital signs will again be recorded every 15 minutes for 1 hour. Additional observations are important particularly in connection with the risk of respiratory depression. These include:

- Nausea and vomiting. This is often due to the nature of the drug being administered.
- Pyrexia indicating presence of infection.
- Level of block. This is usually done by testing sensory function using a block of ice.
- Pain score. Recorded to monitor efficacy. A simple pain chart with a scale of 0–3 is recommended (Davis, 2000):
  0 = no pain
  1 = mild pain
  2 = moderate pain
  3 = severe pain
- Rate of infusion.
- Check catheter site. Needs to be checked at least once each shift to ensure no signs of leakage, secure catheter placement, no kinking of line and no signs of skin irritation or infection.
- Strict fluid balance. Output will be monitored via a urethral catheter. Intravenous access must be maintained at all times whilst an epidural is in progress.

Local policy will indicate when the anaesthetist needs to be informed regarding problems with, level of block, respiration rate, pain score or low systolic blood pressure.

Answer to question two:
Identify the nursing care that Vijay will need during the first 48 hours after his return from theatre.

This period will be an anxious time for both Vijay and his family. The initial part of this period will probably be spent in a high dependency area, depending on local policy and facilities. He will require reassurance and information about all nursing procedures in order to alleviate anxiety and improve compliance with care. It is important that analgesia is effectively maintained in order that Vijay may begin to mobilise and undertake deep breathing exercises and chest physiotherapy in order to reduce the likelihood of post-operative complications.

- Once fully conscious, Vijay should be nursed comfortably in a sitting up position in order to assist breathing (Parboteeah, 1998). He will initially be receiving oxygen therapy. Oxygen saturation levels should be monitored ensuring that the oxygen is delivered at the prescribed rate and by the correct mask or nasal cannulae.
- Frequent observations of blood pressure, pulse, respirations and temperature to identify any complications following surgery, such as haemorrhage and the onset of infection. The frequency of these observations will not only be determined by his condition but also by the length of time that his epidural analgesia is in progress.
- A central venous pressure line will also be in situ and measurements should be recorded.
- Vijay will remain comfortable by receiving adequate analgesia – the observations of which were addressed in the previous question. Epidural analgesia may be administered for about 5–7 days, after which time it may be discontinued, and appropriate alternative analgesics may be given as prescribed. (Mallett & Dougherty (2000).
- An intravenous infusion will be in progress through which he will initially have a blood transfusion (refer to Case 20 for guidelines on Blood transfusion). Observations should be made in order to detect any adverse reaction. As previously stated venous access should be maintained for the duration of the epidural analgesia.
- Vijay will have a naso-gastric tube in situ that should be on free drainage. The amount and type of drainage should be observed and recorded.
- It will be necessary for Vijay to have a urinary catheter in situ. Initially his urine output will need to be measured hourly until his condition stabilises and then the recording can be reduced to 4 hourly. All appropriate catheter care should be given to minimise the risk of him developing a urinary tract infection.
- Vijay will have a large abdominal wound and a tube drain in situ. The wound dressing should be observed for any leakage. The volume and type of drainage from the tube drain should be observed and recorded. Prophylactic antibiotics will be given.
- He will begin gentle mobilising during this period, initially sitting out of bed for short periods. He will continue to wear his anti-embolism stockings

and receive subcutaneous injections of low-molecular heparin. During his time spent in bed he should be encouraged to do leg exercises to reduce the risk of developing deep vein thrombosis.

- As his mobility will be greatly reduced, his risk of developing pressure ulcers should be continually reassessed using a recognised risk assessment tool. His position in bed should be changed at regular intervals whilst observing for any redness over bony prominences. If indicated, he should be nursed on an appropriate pressure relieving mattress.
- Vijay will need assistance with all his hygiene at this time. Mouth care should also be given to counter the drying effect of the oxygen therapy and to make his mouth more comfortable as he will be nil by mouth for about 7–10 days.
- As Vijay will not have anything by mouth for a long period of time, it may be necessary to consider alternative methods of providing nutrition. This will depend on his pre-operative nutritional assessment. He may receive total parenteral nutrition (TPN).

Answer to question three:
What advice and help may be given to Vijay by the multi-disciplinary team to prepare Vijay for his discharge home?

Vijay's progress will be under constant review by the multi-disciplinary team:

- Dietetic advice should be given with supporting leaflets if available. Vijay will have to adapt to eating small amounts of food more often with possibly a change to his diet, avoiding highly spiced foods and perhaps having dietary supplements. He should be advised about any digestive problems that may occur such as dumping syndrome (Torrance & Serginson, 1997). This will also have been raised pre operatively.
- Advice and possible medication to correct any bowel problems. Diarrhoea can be a significant problem following gastrectomy.
- There should be contact with the primary care team (PCT) as Vijay will need to receive vitamin B12 injections (cyanocobalamin) to avoid developing pernicious anaemia. This is as a result of a loss of intrinsic factor, normally produced in the stomach, which is necessary for the absorption of this vitamin (Hallett, 2000).
- Depending on Vijay's histology and prognosis it will probably be necessary for him to receive chemotherapy. He and his family may receive future support from gastrointestinal nurse specialists or Macmillan nurses.
- Prior to discharge Vijay will need a mobility assessment and receive advice about lifting, driving and gradually returning to his normal level of activity.
- A social work referral may be necessary to address any employment issues/concerns Vijay may have.

References

Davis, B. (2000) Routledge essentials for nurses. Caring for People in Pain. London: Routledge.

Hallett, A. (2000) Ch.15. Patients requiring gastrointestinal surgery. In: Pudner, R. (Ed.) Nursing the Surgical Patient. Edinburgh: Bailliere Tindall.

Mallett, J., Dougherty, L. (2000) (Eds) Ch. 15. Epidural analgesia. The Royal Marsden Hospital Manual of Clinical Nursing Procedures. (5th ed.). Oxford: Blackwell Science Ltd.

Parboteeah, S. (1998) Ch. 8. Gastrointestinal Surgery, 168–197. In Simpson, P. (Ed.) Introduction to Surgical Nursing. London: Arnold.

Torrance, C., Serginson, E. (1997) Surgical Nursing. (12th ed.). Edinburgh: Bailliere Tindall.

Additional reading

Chapman, S., Day, R. (2001) Spinal anatomy and the use of epidurals. Professional Nurse 16(6): 1174–1177.

Hicks, S.J. (2001) Gastric cancer: diagnosis, risk factors, treatment and life issues. British Journal of Nursing 10(8): 529–536.

Jacques, A. (1994) Epidural analgesia. British Journal of Nursing 3(14): 734–738.

Useful address

CancerBACUP, 3 Bath Place, Rivington street, London EC2A 3JR or www.cancerbacup.org.uk

First aid

Danny Pertab

> Paul Armitage is a 50-year-old businessman, who frequently commutes long distances. He is separated from his common law wife. He has four grown up children but they do not keep in contact. At weekends he enjoys playing golf and fly fishing.
>
> One autumn evening whilst driving home he is involved in a road traffic accident involving several vehicles and casualties. Paul sustains injuries to his head, chest, abdomen, and lower limbs. He is conscious and responding to pain. Initially he received first aid treatment at the scene of the accident by a passenger in another car who happens to be trained in first aid. Paul's condition was stabilised and he was subsequently airlifted to the nearest Accident and Emergency (A & E) department. On arrival to the hospital Paul showed signs of clinical shock: blood pressure 90/77 mmHg, a weak and thready pulse of 108 beats per minute, shallow breaths and a respiratory rate of 17 per minute. He appeared pale and his extremities were cold. The hospital staff have attempted to contact his relatives, but have so far been unsuccessful.

Question one: Describe the principles of first aid and the role of the first aider.

20 minutes

Question two: Identify the main signs and symptoms of shock that Paul is likely to show.

15 minutes

Question three: Discuss the emergency trauma care that Paul will receive.

30 minutes

Time allowance: **65 minutes**

Answer to question one:
Describe the principles of first aid and the role of the first aider.

The aims of first aid are three fold:

- To preserve life
- To limit worsening of the condition
- To promote healing.

The Voluntary Aid Societies (1999)

The role of a first aider in any accident situation is multifaceted. These include:

- Assessing the situation quickly and safely.
- Protecting casualties and others at the accident from danger.
- Identifying as far as possible the injury or nature of illness affecting a casualty.
- Giving each casualty early and appropriate treatment, treating the most serious first.
- Arranging for the casualty's transfer to hospital, into the care of a doctor, or to his or her home.

The Voluntary Aid Societies (1999)

In a road traffic accident particularly on a busy road, there are many potential dangers such as moving traffic, risk of fire and explosions, spillage of toxic and corrosive substances as well as the potential presence of onlookers. The principle is 'safety first'.

The first aider should identify potential dangers and ensure safety for all concerned. A quick survey of casualties and the severity of their injuries should be assessed to prioritise treatment of those individuals with the most serious conditions. These victims include the unconscious, those who are experiencing severe external bleeding, or breathing problems, the paralysed or even those in a severe panicked state, who need to be handled firmly but with sensitivity. Assistance must be sought immediately from other commuters to assist with the wounded. Whilst waiting for emergency services to arrive, the first aider controls the movement of traffic, coordinates activities of other helpers, attends to those needing essential first aid and monitors their progress. The role of the first aider is by rule completed when they hand over responsibilities to emergency service staff. To minimise the risk of further injuries, Paul should not be moved from the accident site unless absolutely necessary.

Answer to question two:
Identify the main signs and symptoms of shock that Paul is likely to show.

The main signs and symptoms of hypovolaemic shock include:

- Paul's skin will show pallor and cyanosis, feel cold and clammy to touch due to loss of blood circulatory volume and tissue hypoxia. This change in colour will be more pronounced in the nail beds, lips and ear lobe. (Baskett, 1993)
- He will be hypotensive with a systolic blood pressure measuring around 90–100 mmHg or below. (Collins, 2000)
- Paul's pulse rate may be rapid and feel thready on palpation. In severe shock both the blood pressure and pulse rate may become unrecordable.
- He will experience air hunger with respirations becoming laboured, shallow and rapid.
- Other associated signs and symptoms may include thirst, diaphoresis (profuse sweating), oliguria, acute pain from trauma wounds, changes in the level of consciousness due to hypoxia, and elevated level of anxiety. (Edwards, 2001)

Answer to question three:
Discuss the emergency trauma care that Paul will receive.

Hospital care is an integral part in the chain of trauma care. It is a continuation of treatment beginning at the scene of the accident, at the roadside in Paul's case and followed through in the hospital setting.

Emergency trauma care embraces a multi disciplinary team approach. It involves four distinct stages: preparation for reception of trauma victims, primary survey and resuscitation phase (initial assessment and management), secondary survey (further assessment and treatment) and definitive care (Moulton & Yates, 1999). Primary survey and resuscitation embraces the **ABCDE** system where

A = Airway with control of the cervical spine
B = Breathing with oxygen
C = Circulation, with control of external blood loss
D = Disability (neurological status)
E = Exposure with environmental considerations (control of body temperature).

(Hodgetts et al, 1997)

Following the first two stages in the chain of trauma care, Paul's treatment will depend upon his progress and presence of associated injuries and their proper management.

Due to the nature and complexity of his injuries, Paul requires medical and nursing interventions. These will include airway management, assistance with breathing, or even a period of elective ventilation. Full mechanical ventilation will help to maintain adequate oxygen and carbon dioxide levels, pH levels and acid base balance. Arterial blood gas analysis and oxygen saturation will indicate effectiveness of these interventions.

Mechanical ventilation provides the opportunity to administer analgesia for maximum pain relief, rest and comfort, without the fear of respiratory depression or apnoea. Controlled hyperventilation may also induce a hypocapnoeic state, thus inhibiting cerebral vasodilatation, reducing cerebral blood flow, reducing cerebral oedema and preventing an increase in intracranial pressure.

Other areas of care may include: intravenous therapy to replace fluid volume and possibly inotropic support to maintain adequate tissue perfusion and renal function; continuous monitoring of vital functions and neurological status; immobilisation and stabilisation of fractures by splints or traction, observation of fracture site and limbs, and associated wound care. The nurse needs to recognise that Paul will be at risk of complications of being confined to bed. Throughout this traumatic period, Paul will require individualised psychological support.

References

Baskett, P.J.F. (1993) Resuscitation Handbook. (2nd ed.). London: Wolfe.
Collins, T. (2000). Understanding shock. Nursing Standard 14(49) 35–39.
Edwards, S. (2001) Shock types, classifications and explorations of the physiological effects. Emergency Nurse 9(2) 29–38.
Hodgetts, T., Deane, S., Gunning, K. (1997) Trauma Rules. London: BMJ Publishing group.

Moulton, C., Yates, D. (1999) Lecture Notes on Emergency Medicine. (2nd ed.) Oxford: Blackwell Science.

The Voluntary Aid Societies (1999) First Aid Manual, Emergency Procedures for Every one at Home, at Work or at Leisure. London: Dorling Kindersley.

Expressive dysphasia

Penny Tremayne

Monica Adams is a 68-year-old married lady who is transferred from an acute medical ward to a Stroke Unit after having a left cerebral hemisphere infarction. Although Monica has a number of problems such as facial muscle weakness and hemiplegia of her right arm and leg, her major difficulty is expressive dysphasia. Monica's speech is slow, her articulation poor and use of grammar simplified. She can write some words but it depends on her mood. She can get upset, tearful and angry. An ex ward sister, Monica who retired 8 years ago lives in a two bedroom bungalow with her husband Graham.

Graham still works part time at a garden centre, although he plans to retire towards the end of the year, so hopefully in the forthcoming year the couple could move.

Monica and Graham spend a lot of time gardening. They have an adopted grown up son who lives close by with his wife and two sons.

Question one: Explain what is meant by the term expressive dysphasia.

15 minutes

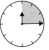

Question two: Outline the nursing interventions that should be offered to Monica with regards to her expressive dysphasia.

30 minutes

Time allowance: **45 minutes**

Client profiles in nursing: adult & the elderly 2

Answer to question one:
Explain what is meant by the term expressive dysphasia.

Expressive dysphasia is a difficulty in the ability to produce speech. Damage to the Broca's area in the speech centre in the brain (Fig. 36.1) means that whilst there is an understanding and even an ability to formulate a logical response in the mind there is a difficulty in articulating the correct words. It presents itself differently in individuals but can result at its most severe with virtual speechlessness, individuals may only be able to say 'yes' or 'no' and these may be used inconsistently and inappropriately (Jackson Anderson, 1996). Individuals can present with what can be described as recurrent utterance where there is the use of a meaningless phrase every time that speech is attempted (Jackson Anderson, 1996). In a less severe form individuals may be able to articulate in key words or short phrases, this is sometimes called telegrammatic speech (Stewart & Creed, 1994). Grammatically there can be errors when speech is produced, verbs and function words often being omitted (Stewart & Creed, 1994, Mohr et al, 1998). At its least severe, individuals with expressive dysphasia can almost speak normally but occasionally have difficult in finding the words required.

In receptive dysphasia there is damage to the Wernicke's area in the speech centre of the brain (Fig. 36.1). In this condition the individual's language as a whole has been drastically reduced, and there can be difficulty in understanding, speaking, reading and writing. The individual may not understand what is being said, or the patient can speak in what can be described as 'tongues', the content meaningless with an absence of grammatical form, words and sounds become mixed up. There can be recurrent utterance where one word is repeated again and again.

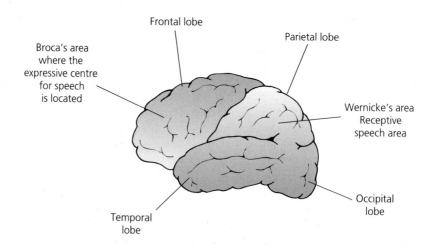

Frontal lobe

Parietal lobe

Broca's area where the expressive centre for speech is located

Wernicke's area Receptive speech area

Occipital lobe

Temporal lobe

Figure 36.1: Speech area in the brain.

Answer to question two:
Outline the nursing interventions that should be offered to Monica with regards to her expressive dysphasia.

One of the most important interventions has already occurred in that Monica is receiving care within a Stroke Unit, early rehabilitative care from such specialist area facilitates improvement and the long term outcome (Department of Health, 2001). Monica will be referred to the Speech and Language Therapy Team who will conduct an individual assessment so that appropriate interventions can be planned. Staff involved in the care of Monica need to be sensitive to the frustration that Monica is going through, in some instances individuals like Monica can experience symptoms of the grieving process (Kubler-Ross, 1970). It is important therefore that staff formulate a quick therapeutic relationship with Monica and her husband so that they can get a better understanding of them and their needs (Stewart & Creed, 1994). Graham should be encouraged to participate in the care of his wife and therefore both of them should be given ongoing explanations of what is happening in relation to interventions and why. Staff need to have an enhanced self awareness when caring for Monica, intellectual capacity is unimpaired and therefore they should adopt appropriate body language and be non judgemental. Body language should be open and interventions should not be rushed. When speaking to Monica, staff should be in her line of vision and speak slowly, using short phrases in simple easily audible, non patronising language. Monica may tire easily and therefore the nurse should keep conversation short. As Monica's attention span may be short it is important to indicate the intention to communicate so that Monica can pay due attention. Should Monica have dentures then it should be ensured that these are well fitting, and if she has a hearing aid this should be in use and fully functional.

The environment surrounding Monica when she is attempting to communicate should be as relaxed as possible with minimal disturbance and distraction (Smith, 1991). According to Jackson Anderson (1996) language should be stimulated by visual or auditory means. To elicit a response cues should be used, for example to stimulate the finding of the word bed, a cue such as 'Bed,............you lie in a _ _ _', should be used. Such an approach avoids the potential of meaningless repetition (Jackson Anderson, 1996). Other suggested stimulating exercises can include 'say what you are wearing', and 'what time is it?' (Eaton Griffith et al, 1996). Smith (1991) considers that staff can use facial expression and gesture to reinforce meaning of words appropriately. Different, relevant methods of communication should be explored in an attempt to ignite interest in a conversation, this can include word and picture charts, writing, song, gesture, drawing, facial expression, touch, magazines, family photographs, postcards, illustrated books, games and quizzes (Smith, 1991; Eaton Griffith et al, 1996). When Monica becomes upset and cannot find the words to what she is trying to say, then staff should try to interpret what she is trying to convey, if this does not work then she should be encouraged to write slowly and clearly so that she can be understood (Stewart & Creed, 1994). Staff should avoid trying to finish off what Monica is trying to say, instead be honest and state to Monica that it is not understood, but could she repeat it, or alternatively

Client profiles in nursing: adult & the elderly 2

write it down. Praise and encouragement should be given to Monica as should the call bell system be explained and readily available to her throughout her rehabilitation.

It must be recognised that the process of rehabilitation is a lengthy one and there will be peaks and troughs during which Monica, her relatives, nursing staff and members of the multi disciplinary team could support each other.

References

Department of Health (2001) National Service Framework for Older People: Modern Standards and Service Models. London: The Stationery Office.

Eaton Griffith, V., Oetliker, P., Oswin, P. (1996) 'A Time to Speak': Positive ideas for Helping Stroke Patients with Speech Problems at Home and in Groups. London: The Stroke Association.

Jackson Anderson, S. (1996) Ch. 4. 'Speech therapy'. In: Johnstone, M. (1996) Home Care for the Stroke Patient: Living in a Pattern. (3rd ed.). Edinburgh: Churchill Livingstone.

Kubler-Ross, E. (1970) On Death and Dying. London: Tavistock Publications.

Mohr, J., Lazar, R., Marshall, R., Gautier, J., Hier, D. (1998) Ch. 19. 'Middle Cerebral Artery Disease'. In: Barnett, H., Mohr, J., Stein, B., Yatsu, F. Stroke: Pathophysiology, Diagnosis, and Management. (3rd ed.). New York: Churchill Livingstone.

Smith, M. (1991) Understanding speech disorders. Nursing Standard 5(48): 30–33.

Stewart, J., Creed, J. (1994) Aphasia: a care study. British Journal of Nursing 3(3): 226–229.

Further reading

Easton, K. (1994) Distinct probabilities. Rehabilitation Nursing 19(5): 303–304.

Scott, A. (2000) Stroke rehabilitation: the role of the nurse. Nursing Times Clinical Monographs No 45. London: NT Books Emap Healthcare Ltd.

Warlow, C., Dennis, M., van Gijn, J., Sandercock, P., Bamford, J., Wardlow, J. (1996) Stroke: A Practical Guide to Management. Oxford: Blackwell Science.

Useful address

The Stroke Association
Stroke House
Whitecross Street
London
EC1Y 8JJ
Tel: 0171 566 0300
Website: www.stroke.org.uk

Last offices

Chris Buswell

The following profile details the laying out of a body in a nursing home. There are no questions to this profile, but readers may wish to use this chapter to reflect on their own experiences and feelings surrounding patients' deaths in their respective workplaces. If you are reading this case and, like Carol the care assistant in the scenario, have not yet encountered a patient's death nor assisted in last offices you may find it useful to write down your feelings and thoughts before reading the scenario. After reading the scenario readers may find it beneficial to re-visit their thoughts and reflect on their feelings surrounding death. Other readers may find it helpful to compare and contrast the differences in last offices between those in the scenario and in their own workplaces. Particular attention should be placed on reading your work-place policies and procedures regarding last offices, coroner's cases, deaths 24 hours after hospital admission or surgery, and also differing religious and cultural needs. The reading list that follows the scenario can provide further opportunities to learn about these aspects in the care of a deceased patient.

Mr Gregory Lauder was an 84-year-old widower. Sadly he has just died peacefully in the nursing home where he spent the last 2 years of his life. Nurse Dawn and care assistant Carol were with Mr Lauder as he passed away. Dawn is explaining to Carol what they are about to do. Carol has been caring for 6 months and has never seen a dead body before:

'I'm just popping this pillow under Mr Lauder's chin to support his jaw so that his mouth stays closed. When his son travels down from Dundee to pay his last respects to his father he'll look more peaceful with a jaw that's closed. When I saw my first dead body, as a student nurse, it was in the hospital chapel of rest. All I could keep looking at was a half opened mouth. It looked so unsightly and macabre. Although the undertakers can get jaws to close by suturing the lips together I think we can help our patients by doing this small thing for them. Some nurses tie a piece of bandage around the dead patient's chin and head to keep the mouth closed but I always think it looks more dignified to have a pillow under the chin, especially in the nursing home in case a family member walks into the room without finding one of us first. Also the bandage may leave pressure marks on Mr Lauder's skin. We'll just straighten out his arms and legs. Although rigor mortis won't set in for at least another 4 hours he'll look more comfortable and dignified. I'll also close his eyes for him. Oh dear this eyelid won't stay shut. Could you pop out and get some vaseline for me please Carol?'

When Carol had left the room Dawn took Mr Lauder's hand and said, 'I know you weren't a religious man Gregory, but I'm going to say a prayer for you.' Dawn closed her eyes and said a quick silent prayer. Opening her eyes again she said, 'You'd probably call me a daft old so and so, but I'm going to miss you, I know how much you've missed your wife and I hope you'll be together again.' As she finished speaking Carol walked back into the room with the vaseline.

'Who were you talking to?' asked Carol.

'Only to Mr Lauder, I know he's dead but I still think of him as a person, rather than just a dead body. Thanks for getting the vaseline.' Dawn put a small amount under his eyelid and closed the eye. 'That should help his eyes stay closed. There he looks like he's asleep, doesn't he?'

'Yes,' said Carol stroking Mr Lauder's arm, 'he's still warm too.'

'I know that Mr Lauder is the first dead person you've seen Carol.'

'Yes he is, but in a way I'm glad that he is. I've known him for 6 months and he was the first patient I'd ever washed. He put me at my ease. He was so funny and the stories about when he was a prisoner of war really opened my eyes. Although he suffered he told me that he forgave the Japanese and got on with his life. Now he's taught me that there's nothing to be frightened about dead people. He really does look peaceful and asleep.'

'Out of respect for Mr Lauder we'll leave him for about an hour,' said Dawn. 'I believe that this gives the spirit enough time to look down at the body and to say goodbye before going on its way. That's why I'm opening the window. It gives the spirit an opportunity to go to the next world. Some nurses believe the spirit may stay for longer and floats above the body, watching what happens.' Dawn finished closing the window and drew the curtains. As she walked back to Carol she touched her shoulder and said, 'Why don't I go and telephone Mr Lauder's son, the doctor and matron while you get yourself a cup of tea and we'll give Mr Lauder a bit of privacy before we come back to wash him.'

Dawn knocked on Mr Lauder's door and entered. 'Hello Mr Lauder, Carol and I have just come to give you a wash before you go to the undertakers. I've telephoned Stuart and he'll visit you there to say goodbye.'

Dawn brought a bowl of soapy water, towel and flannel and put them down on Mr Lauder's bedside table. Carol and Dawn put on a pair of gloves and an apron. Unconsciously Carol looked first at Mr Lauder and then above him.

'You know Carol, some nurses don't wash dead patients, especially if they go straight to the undertakers, but I like to do this. It's a good way of showing our respects and saying goodbye. I think it's important for all the staff on duty to say goodbye because we do get quite attached to our patients in nursing homes. We see them day in day out, meet their family regularly and hear all about their past. It's quite a privilege really.'

Dawn notices that Carol is hesitant to wash Mr Lauder and starts to wash his face whilst talking to Mr Lauder, explaining what she is doing. 'When you last touched Mr Lauder he felt warm, but now that blood is no longer circulating around him he'll feel a bit cooler and have blotchy, waxy skin. That's perfectly normal. Why don't you dry his face for him Carol?' asked Dawn as she gently handed the towel to Carol.

Carol at first gingerly dried Mr Lauder's face and was soon confidently helping Dawn to wash Mr Lauder, shave him and clean his dentures. However as Carol and Dawn rolled Mr Lauder onto his side he groaned.

'God,' cried Carol as she sprang back in fright, 'he's still alive.'

'No he's not,' smiled Dawn as she gently eased Mr Lauder onto his back. 'That noise was just the release of trapped air from Mr Lauder's lungs. Some people think of it as the last breath the dying person took finally being released by the body. Some bodies will give a gentle sigh, others a large grunt. Don't worry I jumped higher than you when it first happened to me!'

Carol gave an embarrassed but relieved sigh and stepped forward to once again assist Dawn. They then put a large continence pad and underpants on Mr Lauder so that if there was any leakage of body fluids they could be absorbed safely, without posing any health hazard to anyone handling the body, before putting him into his clean pyjamas. 'He looks so much better after a wash, change of clothes and a hair brush,' said Carol.

'Yes he does, doesn't he? When I last worked in a hospital we had to dress our dead patients in horrible paper shrouds with ties at the back. They looked awful. Then we had to wrap the body in a sheet and stick a label on the sheet with the person's details. We'd also have to ensure the patient had an identification label on their wrist and ankle. It seemed so clinical, but it did help the mortuary staff to identify the bodies and prevent any health hazards to the porters. I used to get a flower from a patient's vase and put it on the body after I'd wrapped it in a sheet. At least Mr Lauder leaves the home with a bit of respect. We'll just cover him over with a sheet and leave his face and an arm exposed. Then if any of the other patients or staff want to say goodbye to him they can talk to him or hold his hand. One care assistant I worked with in another nursing home always had a lavender scented candle in her locker. If someone died on her shift she'd come to say goodbye to the person and light the candle and leave it burning until the body left the nursing home. We'll go back to the nursing station and check Mr Lauder's care plan. There may be some details of predeath wishes or a preference to a specific undertaker. Some patients or their families do pre-pay and arrange funerals. I'll write Mr Lauder's details out for the undertakers. Remind me to write on the form that we've left Mr Lauder wearing his wedding ring. His son can decide whether he wants his dad to keep it on. I'll also have to mention Mr Lauder's pacemaker. The undertakers will have to arrange to remove this if Mr Lauder is to be cremated since its battery will cause an explosion. Undertakers also need to know if the patient had a hip replacement for the same reason. We can list all his valuables and belongings later and pack them up for Stuart, I'm sure he'll appreciate us doing that after his journey down. His son will be relieved that dad won't need a post mortem because his death was expected and Mr Lauder saw his general practitioner this morning. If Mr Lauder had died within 24 hours of being admitted to the home or a hospital, or had died suddenly and unexpectedly, or if it was suspected that he died from the result of an industrial disease such as mesothelioma then he would have had to have a post mortem and probably be referred to the Coroner's. The same goes for anyone who dies within 24 hours of surgery. The local policy in this area is that anyone not seen by a doctor in the last 2 weeks must have a post mortem. By not needing a post mortem there will be less stress and upset for Mr Lauder's son and the funeral won't be delayed'

As Carol and Dawn leave the room Carol whispered, 'Goodbye Mr Lauder and God Bless.'

Suggested further reading

Black, J. (1991) Death and bereavement: the customs of Hindus, Sikhs and Moslems. Bereavement Care 10(1): 6–8.
Braun, K., Pietsch, J., Blanchette, P. (2000) (Eds) Cultural Issues in End Of Life Decision Making. London: Sage.

Buswell, C. (1998) The right to grieve. Elderly Care 10(3): 20–21.

Cobb, M. (2001) The Dying Soul: Spiritual Care at the End of Life. Buckingham: Open University Press.

Cooke, H. (2000) When Someone Dies. Oxford: Butterworth Heinemann.

Crummey, V. (1997) Major undertaking. Nursing Times 93(11): 72–78.

Green, J., Green, M. (1992) Dealing with Death: Practices and Procedures. London: Chapman and Hall.

Hinnells, J. (1996) A Handbook of Living Religions. (2nd ed.). Oxford: Blackwells.

Mallett, J., Dougherty, L. (2000) (Eds) The Royal Marsden Hospital Manual of Clinical Nursing Procedures. (5th ed.). Oxford: Blackwell Science, pp 345–354.

Nearney, L. (1998) Last offices, part one. Nursing Times 94(26): 2 unnumbered pages.

Nearney, L. (1998) Last offices, part two. Nursing Times 94(27): 2 unnumbered pages.

Nearney, L. (1998) Last offices, part three. Nursing Times 94(28): 2 unnumbered pages.

Neuberger, J. (1992) Caring for Dying People of Different Faiths. (2nd ed.). London: Mosby.

Neuberger, J. (1999) Dying Well: A Guide to Enabling a Good Death. Hale: Hochland and Hochland.

Nyatanga, B. (1997) Cultural issues in palliative care. International Journal of Palliative care 3(4): 203–208.

Sander, R., Russell, P. (2001) Care for dying people in nursing homes. Nursing Older People 13(2): 21–24.

Speck, P. (1992) Care after death. Nursing Times 88(6): 20.

Coventry University